GREAT

REDUCED CANCER!

2nd Edition

A scientific approach

to great sleep and reduced risk of cancer

Richard L. Hansler Ph.D.

ISBN: 1500231371
ISBN 13: 9781500231378
Library of Congress Control Number: 2014911241
CreateSpace Independent Publishing Platform,
North Charleston, South Carolina

DEDICATION

This book is dedicated to those who are at high risk for cancer and for whom the ideas in this book may offer some increased hope.

ACKNOWLEDGEMENTS

Thanks go first of all to my wife, Wanda, for her patience and support while I try to spread the word about the benefits of melatonin. Next, I need to thank my partners in this venture, Dr. Ed Carome, Vilnis Kubulins and Dr. Marty Alpert. It continues to be great fun trying to make this academic study into a business that helps people. Many on the faculty and staff at John Carroll University have been extremely helpful in so many ways. Dr. Joe Trivisonno, Dr. Sally Wertheim, Dr. Joe Miller, Dr. Mary Beadle, Dr. Roy Day, Ms. Diega Bravo, Ms. Carol Clark and Ms. Tonya Strong-Charles. I also want to thank and acknowledge the support of dear friends, Dr. Mike and Mary Michael. I also want to thank the thirty-some students who worked in the Lighting Innovations Institute over the past 12 years for the inspiration they have provided. I also want to thank my colleague and friend from my years at GE, John Davenport. It was his vision that was behind my move to JCU after retirement. I need to thank and acknowledge the important role that Rev. Dick and Susie Sering have played in my life. Their complete commitment to helping others has been an inspiration to thousands. In Dick's many-year fight against cancer he inspired me to continue a search for a way to overcome that menace to the health of so many. I also want to thank my children and grandchildren for their love and support that have helped to create the climate where I have been able to continue working well past normal retirement age.

INTRODUCTION

The first edition of *Great Sleep! Reduced Cancer!* was published in 2008 and the second in 2014. Because the newer studies still support the ideas presented in the first edition, the first part of this book consists of the text of the first edition, without any changes. If you have already read it, you can skip right to the second half. If you have not read it, please do so before going to the second half. My idea is to keep the same format in the second half and simply expand on the ideas and present the results of the recent studies.

In the second half of this book, the chapters are numbered the same as the chapters in the first edition but with an *A* added; the titles have otherwise been kept the same. Some readers may want to read the first edition of a given chapter and then read the second edition of the same chapter. In any event, I hope you enjoy reading this book. It might save your life.

TABLE OF CONTENTS

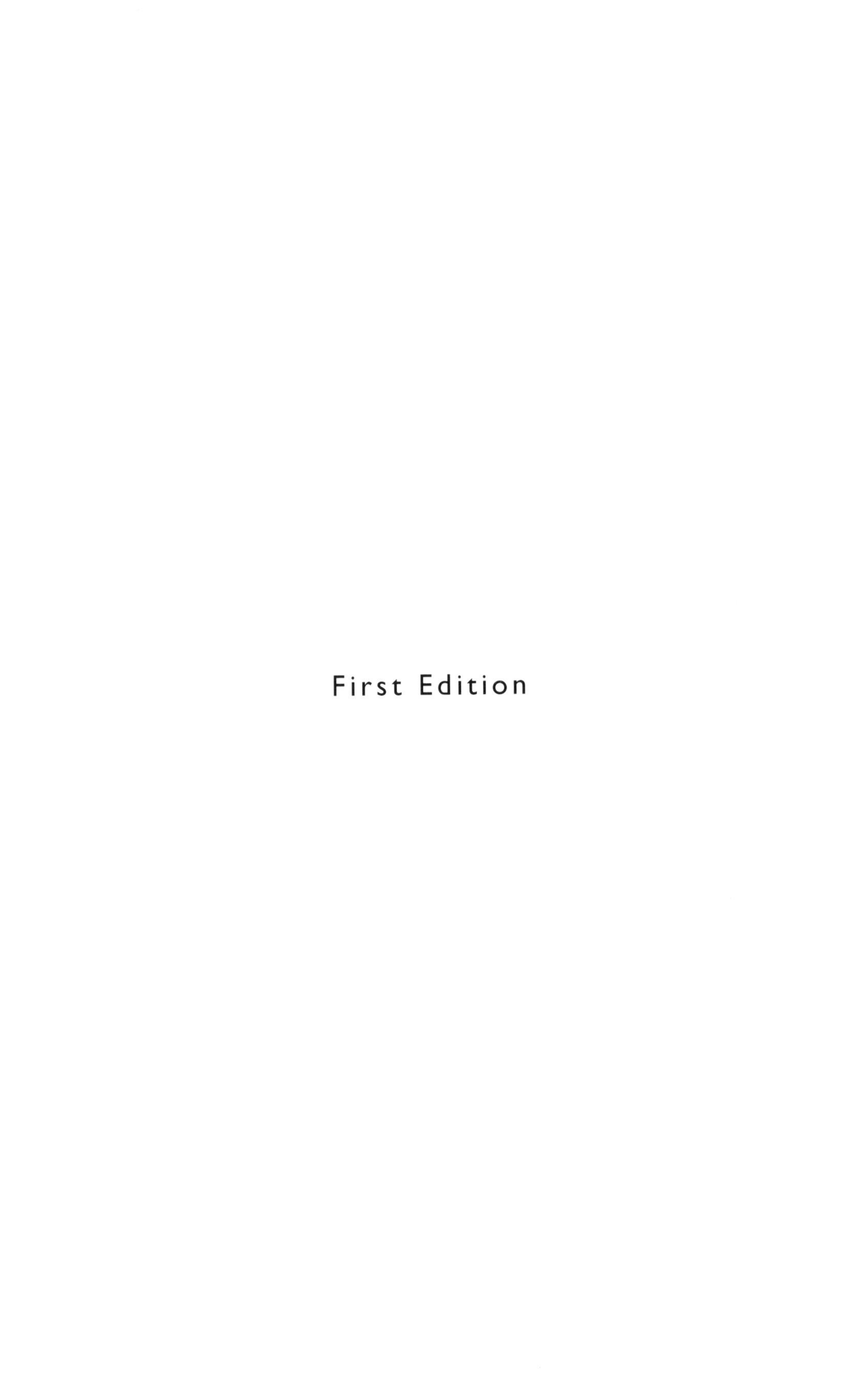

First Edition

PREFACE

In December 2007, the International Agency for Cancer Research (IARC) that is part of the World Health Organization (WHO) determined that shift work is a "probable cause of cancer." This is one more step in a series of warnings from the scientific community that began in 1987 when Richard Stevens published what is now called the "melatonin hypothesis." It is the belief that the loss of the cancer-fighting hormone melatonin when the eyes are exposed to light during the night is partly responsible for the rise in the cancer rate that has occurred in industrial countries.

Here is the verbatim statement from IARC:

> **Shift work that involves circadian disruption is "probably carcinogenic to humans"**
>
> *Epidemiological studies have found that long-term nightworkers have a higher risk of breast cancer than women who do not work at night. These studies have involved mainly nurses and flight attendants. The studies are consistent with animal studies that demonstrate that constant light, dim light at night, or simulated chronic jet lag can substantially increase tumour development. Other experimental studies show that reducing melatonin levels at night increases the incidence or growth of tumours.*
>
> *These results may be explained by the disruption of the circadian system that is caused by exposure to light at night. This can alter sleep-activity patterns, suppress melatonin production, and disregulate genes involved in tumour development. Among the many different patterns of shiftwork, those that include nightwork are most disruptive to the circadian system.*
>
> *"Nearly 20% of the working population in Europe and North America is engaged in shiftwork, which is most prevalent in the health-care,*

industrial, transportation, communications, and hospitality sectors. To date, most studies have focused on breast cancer in nurses and flight attendants. Now more studies are needed to examine this potential risk in other professions and for other cancers," noted Dr. Cogliano, head of the IARC Monographs Programme.

End of statement from IARC.

It is unfortunate that this warning from WHO suggests that if you are not a shift worker that this is not of interest to you. It is the purpose of this book to document why using light at night is a problem for everyone. We will not only spell out the problem but provide a number of practical ways to deal with it.

While reducing the risk of cancer is a high priority, there are many other ways in which using light at night impacts health. The factor that connects the various conditions that benefit from controlling light at night is melatonin and its many effects on the body, including sleep and body temperature. Conditions as diverse as Seasonally Affective Disorder (SAD), Attention Deficit Hyperactivity Disorder (ADHD), Fibromyalgia/chronic fatigue syndrome, bipolar disorder, and postpartum depression all respond to controlling light.

While treating these serious conditions by controlling light is important and rewarding, the most broadly significant result of controlling light at night is the improvement in the quality of sleep experienced by so many people. If this were the only benefit, it would be of great value, especially to those who have suffered from poor quality of sleep for many years.

INTRODUCTION

I started writing this book a year ago when it seemed that the most important thing to do was to warn people about the use of light at night and how it increases the risk of cancer, as well as to let them know there was a way to avoid the problem. The circumstantial evidence continues to mount that cancer can be caused by the use of light in the hours before bedtime. That's really not the right way to say it. The light itself does not cause the cancer. All kinds of other things, like radiation, toxins, mutations, etc., cause cancer cells to be formed. Using light at night prevents the body from producing its own defenders that will kill the cancer cells. Despite the presence of a large body of evidence supporting this view, the only way the medical profession will believe it is if a very large clinical trial proves it beyond a shadow of doubt.

People at high risk for cancer don't have to wait until the clinical trials are complete to take appropriate action. They can examine the evidence themselves at places like www.PubMed.gov. That's a wonderful website maintained by the U.S. government that abstracts medical papers as fast as they are published. It has a terrific search engine that seems to know what you want. People can put in the words "cancer light melatonin" and the search engine will turn up abstract after abstract of technical papers from all over the world that document the evidence.

Those at high risk for cancer will likely decide that using light at night is something they need to be concerned about. Information on what to do about it is less readily available. This is why I am writing this book. The media are not a lot different from the medical profession. They don't want to alarm people if the problem isn't real. They all have their editorial boards, which usually include representatives of the medical profession. One can ask, "Where were they during the smoking and cancer controversy?" While not completely analogous to the tobacco situation, there are some parallels. It can take years before a cancer develops to where it is easily detected. There are vested interests in the form of big companies making money from the products. In this case, it's the whole lighting industry.

Experts don't all agree there is a problem or, if there is, that it is a serious problem. One obvious difference between this problem and smoking is that one can quit smoking. Giving up the use of light at night just isn't going to happen. Fortunately that isn't required.

CHAPTER 1.

Cutting the Risk of Cancer

I won't hold the readers in suspense just to keep them reading. The answer of how to reduce the risk of cancer by 50% or more is contained in a press release issued in March 2006. It is available to anyone who can find it. Did the *New York Times* pick it up and publish it? Are you kidding? Hardly anyone did. I'll reprint it here.

> *University Heights, OH (PRWEB) March 8, 2006 – Blind people have about half the risk of cancer as people with normal vision according to a large study by the National Health Service. The most likely reason is that they produce melatonin and other secretions from the pineal gland for 9 or 10 hours a night while the rest of us only make them for 6 or 7 hours a night. Melatonin is a powerful cancer fighter, but the body only makes it when in the dark. Exposing the eyes to light shuts down the pineal gland.*
>
> *But there is good news. Not all colors of light cause melatonin suppression. It's only the blue rays that cause the problem. This means that blocking the blue light from entering the eye the pineal gland can continue making melatonin. Glasses that block blue light are available at www.lowbluelights.com.*
>
> *The fact that blind people only have half the rate of cancer was first discovered in the '90s and has been confirmed by more recent studies. A related study of women who consistently sleep unusually long found that the incidence of breast cancer for women who slept 9 hours or more a night was only about one fourth that of women who*

slept 6 or 7 hours a night. A subsequent study found that women who slept unusually long made melatonin for a similarly unusually long time.

Concern about the use of light at night began when it was found that nurses who worked night shift from time to time had a higher incidence of breast cancer. Something about disrupting the circadian rhythm of the body was causing a higher risk of cancer. Studies in animals show that continuous exposure to light accelerates the rate of growth of cancerous tumors. The mechanism is thought to be the lack of melatonin.

Last fall the results of a milestone study were published. The response of human breast cancers to blood with and without pineal secretions was studied. Breast cancers grew rapidly when exposed to blood without melatonin but only very slowly when the blood contained melatonin. Dr. Blask who led the study said that "Melatonin puts the cancer to sleep at night." Unfortunately exposing the eyes to light at night wakes up the cancer and lets it grow rapidly.

Wearing glasses that block the blue light for a few hours before going to bed lets people regain the long hours of melatonin flow that is experienced by blind people. The glasses allow the yellow, orange and red light to pass through so one can read, watch television or work on a computer with no problem. Users of the glasses also report a marked improvement in sleep, which supports the idea that more melatonin is being produced. This minor change in life style could cut cancer risk in half.

So now that you know the answer about what you need to do to reduce your risk of cancer, you can close the book and go on with your life. That is an option, but I encourage you to read on. It turns out that the same idea of avoiding blue light at night has many more benefits—benefits we didn't realize we had when Edison unveiled his first big invention, the incandescent light bulb.

For the skeptics that want to examine the evidence that using light at night increases the risk of cancer, we will do just that in Chapter 17.

CHAPTER 2.

Light and Sleep

Light has always been considered synonymous with beauty, goodness, and health. For example, we talk about a healthy glow, heavenly light, basking in sunlight. Darkness has always been associated with evil; for example, the devil is often called the prince of darkness.

Windsor P. Hall wrote, "The equivalence of light and goodness is witnessed in every aspect of society: it is referenced in literature, art, film, and even by parents when they wisely admonish, 'Nothing good happens late at night.' Perhaps the symbolism of light and dark has such a prominent role in our psyche because it carries a connotation that cannot be removed: it is universally and inevitably understood that light, with its warmth and energy, brings health and prosperity to all living things. Thus, light is good in both the literal and figurative sense, and this concept dominates the human perception of life."

In Genesis we learn that "God separated the light from the darkness and he called the light day and the darkness he called night. And God saw the light and it was good." Jesus called himself, "The light of the world." Without the continuous light from the sun, life on earth would soon end.

When human life evolved, up to the time that fire was discovered, there was only the natural light from the sun, moon, and stars. All the early forms of artificial light—the torch, the candle, and the gas flame—were all just a form of fire. It's only been for about one hundred years that we have had truly artificial light; that is, light that is not really from a fire.

The early days of artificial light employed the carbon filament, which wasn't all that much hotter than a flame. It wasn't until the invention of the tungsten filament that really high temperature light sources arrived. The carbon arc has temperatures rivaling the surface of the sun. The mercury arc, high-pressure sodium lamps, fluorescent lamps, and metal halide lamps all produce light much different than the light from a fire or a candle.

What is it about these more recent artificial lights that is so different from the light sources under which we evolved? The main difference lies in the amount of blue wavelengths present in the light from these sources. There is a great deal of evidence that it is this blue light from these newer sources that is causing many of the health problems in modern society.

In the parts of the earth near the equator there are twelve hours of daylight and twelve hours of darkness, year round. Because the earth is tipped at an angle to the plane of its orbit around the sun, the parts of the earth away from the equator experience longer days during the summer and shorter days in the winter. However, on average over the whole year, we still get twelve hours of daylight and twelve hours of darkness. For the past hundred years we have extended the hours of daylight with our artificial lights. The typical American sleeps less than seven hours a night and spends only that amount of time in darkness. The rest of the twenty-four hours, (seventeen hours) is spent in light. In this book we will be examining what we know about the effect on the human body of this big change in exposure to light.

Insomnia has been around forever, yet there are a number of signs that it is becoming more common. The first chapter in the Bible describes how Jacob had trouble sleeping: "Thus I was; by day the heat consumed me, and the cold by night, and my **sleep** fled from my eyes." Even the idea of reading when you can't sleep goes back to biblical times. "On that night the king could not **sleep**; and he gave orders to bring the book of memorable deeds, the chronicles, and they were read before the king."

Shakespeare is thought to have suffered from insomnia based on the number of characters in his plays who had trouble sleeping. Franklin H. Head has written a whole book on the subject, *Shakespeare's Insomnia and the Causes Thereof.* Ben Franklin also had trouble sleeping. He was of the opinion that the temperature of his bed was very important. If he couldn't sleep, he would get up and wait for his bed to cool down before trying to sleep again. Napoleon planned his conquests during the nights he couldn't sleep. Edison slept only a short time during the night but would take naps during the day.

Polls of the American people indicate that about half of those who are asked whether they sleep well will reply "no!" The number of medical doctors who are specially trained to treat sleep disorders has risen dramatically. The number of papers published in scientific journals that deal with sleep medicine has risen from almost zero in the 1940s to over 1,100 in the first five years of this century. Between 1990 and 2000 the number of papers dealing with insomnia doubled. The National Sleep Foundation estimates sleeping problems cost this country $100 billion a year in lost productivity, accidents, and medical bills.

As with most of the problems in our modern world, we look to solve our poor sleeping habits with a quick fix. If we can't sleep, we take a pill to fix it. The pharmaceutical industry has been quick to respond to our needs. It seems every month brings an announcement of a new and better sleeping pill. While pills may have a place in treating sleep disorders, it would seem to make sense to try to understand the basis of the problem.

Much of this problem of getting a good night's sleep is blamed on stress associated with our hectic lifestyle. While this is no doubt a factor in poor sleep, the thesis of this book is that there is a more prevalent source of the problem associated with our modern society: the use of artificial light. Before Edison, humans had mostly the sun to provide light. Now, everywhere we go we have brightly lit surroundings, including our ever larger and brighter TV screens and our ubiquitous computers. Even outdoors at night we can't escape light. The sky is so bright from the street lights and signs that it is hard to see more than the brightest stars.

What is it about light that might explain our poor sleep? It's the same thing that is increasing our risk of cancer. It's been known for many years that light suppresses the production of the sleep hormone melatonin. It is called a sleep hormone because it makes us feel drowsy when it is present in our bloodstream. To understand how this happens, we need to examine how light striking our eyes controls the production of melatonin.

The pineal gland is a tiny gland located at the base of the brain near the center of the head. It is about the size of a pea, shaped like a pine cone (hence the name), yet is one of the most important parts of the human body. It is so important that there is a technical journal, "Journal of Pineal Research," devoted entirely to papers about this organ. Nerve fibers run from the retina of the eye, by a somewhat complicated path, to the pineal gland. Nearby is the body's internal or circadian clock that provides the body with a schedule of waking and sleeping. Light plays an important role in setting this clock. There is increasing evidence that all of the cells in the body experience a circadian rhythm, with the secretions of the pineal gland keeping them all in phase.

Melatonin is the main hormone produced by the pineal gland. There are melatonin receptors located in many places throughout the body that are activated when melatonin is present in the blood. The circadian clock will cause the pineal gland to start producing melatonin, but only if the eyes are in darkness or in very dim light. The time when this happens is the most reliable method of knowing how the circadian clock is set. It is so important in sleep research it is abbreviated as DLMO (dim light melatonin onset). If one is in darkness or dim light, the melatonin will begin to flow at the same time each evening. This melatonin signal travels to all parts of the body and keeps all the parts of the body in synchronization.

What happens if, instead of being in dim light when DLMO should be happening, the eyes are exposed to bright light? If the light is on for only an hour or two, it will simply delay the start of the melatonin flow. If it is quite bright and persists throughout the night, the light will completely suppress melatonin production. If the light is present every evening for a few hours, it will push back the DLMO to the time when the light is normally extinguished; that is, it will reset the circadian clock. The circadian clock is not reset easily. Anyone who has experienced jet lag knows it takes about a week to recover from a time change of six hours such as is typical on a trip to Europe.

Recent studies have begun to indicate that there are really two internal clocks: one that initiates the flow of melatonin and a second one that controls shutting it off. A really strange aspect of the whole situation is that not only does light control the clocks, but melatonin itself plays a role in setting the clocks. Blind people typically have a free-running circadian clock. That means it may not be in step with the clock on the wall. It may not be turning on melatonin production during the nighttime when the person would like to sleep. Since light won't work with blind people in setting the circadian clock, melatonin has been tried. Giving a small amount by mouth at the same time every evening has been successful in entraining the circadian clock to the blind person's sleep schedule.

Part of the problem in sleeping arises when people keep changing their daily schedule. The circadian clock will let the body know it's 11:00 p.m., time to go to bed, but if we stay up till 2:00 a.m., the next night the circadian clock may not start making melatonin till nearly midnight. Experiments with animals show that if the schedule is continuously changed, soon the pineal gland will be producing very little melatonin.

Going into darkness each evening at a regular time is important for keeping melatonin flowing. What happens in the morning is also important. Exposing the eyes to light at a regular time each morning is at least as important as what happens in the evening. What happens in the evening seems to have the biggest impact on the circadian clock that controls the start of the melatonin flow. What happens in the morning seems to impact both the clock that starts melatonin flow and the one that turns it off. Keeping a reasonably regular time both to retire and arise is one key to a good night's sleep. It's not important when you go to bed or get out of bed but what time you go into darkness in the evening and when your eyes receive light in the morning.

You will see in the next chapter why it's not just how much light is required, but the color of the light that determines how the pineal gland responds. How much the melatonin flow is suppressed by light depends on the intensity, the color, and the duration of the exposure. It also depends to some extent on the previous exposure to light. If the individual has been in dim light for a long time, a larger response will occur.

In summary, there are two internal clocks that start and stop the flow of melatonin at the same time every day if the individual is in darkness. The natural period of flow is nine or ten hours, if the individual remains in darkness that long. Light causes the pineal gland to shut down or not start making melatonin. Keeping a regular schedule of light and darkness improves the quality of sleep. An irregular schedule results in less melatonin and poorer sleep.

CHAPTER 3.

The Remarkable Discovery That Blue Light Suppresses Melatonin

Dr. George Brainard is a professor at Thomas Jefferson University who has studied melatonin production in animals and humans for many years. He knew that light suppressed melatonin production but began to wonder if the color of the light was important. He set up a huge experiment in which volunteers stared into a sphere lit with light of just one color and then were tested for the level of melatonin in their blood. A few days later the experiment was repeated with a different color. This was done with a large number of volunteers and the data averaged.

The result was very interesting. The blue light had the biggest effect in suppressing melatonin, with a peak at a particular wavelength (470nm). This did not agree with the corresponding measurements for either the rods or the cones that are responsible for vision. These are apparently a new type of sensor. A similar test was going on in the U.K. at the University of Surrey with identical results. The timekeeping function of the body (circadian clock) appears to have little or no connection to the visual system.

These historic findings were not published until 2001 in simultaneous papers. It's quite amazing that such a basic fact about the eyes had escaped detection throughout the twentieth century.

This finding is the whole basis for this book. In it lies the key to great sleep. It means that if we block blue light from entering the eye, the pineal gland will perform in exactly the same way as if the eyes were in darkness. By putting on glasses that block the blue light a couple of hours before bedtime, melatonin will begin to flow. When bedtime arrives, the amount of melatonin will be quite large, so the individual will fall asleep very quickly and sleep soundly. In this way, the full nine or ten hours of melatonin flow will be obtained.

A subsequent study by Brainard to the groundbreaking discovery that blue light is responsible for melatonin suppression was a 2003 study in which the sensitivity of the inferior (lower) and superior (upper) parts of the retina were compared. If only the superior part was illuminated, the response was no different than if the eyes were in darkness. When the inferior portion was illuminated with 200 lux of white light for ninety minutes, the melatonin was significantly suppressed. This could be interpreted to mean the blue of the sky was the source of the light that informed the body it was daytime. One could argue that this is why the sensors respond most strongly to blue light.

Another interesting result of more recent studies of suppression of melatonin by light exposure is the discovery by Ruger in 2005. He found that the nasal portion of the retina is much more sensitive to the light that controls melatonin than the temporal part. In the experiments, the different portions of the retina were exposed to 100 lux of white light for four hours. Exposure of the nasal portion resulted in immediate suppression of melatonin and a shift of seventy-eight minutes in the circadian rhythm. The same exposure to the temporal portion resulted in much less suppression and no shift in the circadian rhythm.

In addition to the importance of exposing the eyes to light in the morning, some recently obtained evidence suggests that exposing the eyes to light in the late afternoon and early evening is also important. In these studies it was demonstrated that the amount of melatonin produced during the following night was increased after exposure to bright light in the afternoon and evening. It was also found that the temperature minimum during the night was lower following exposure to bright light during the day before. The depth of the core temperature drop of the human body is thought to be a good measure of the quality of sleep. Studies in nursing homes showed the residents were more alert during the day and slept more soundly at night when there was a high level of light during the day.

This may be part of the reason that using the glasses in the evening does not appear to help all those who have tried them to treat insomnia. If the patients are not getting enough light to completely suppress melatonin during the day and evening, putting on the glasses would not be expected to make any difference. Perhaps the first approach to insomnia is to try bright light during the day before trying to block ambient light in the time before bedtime.

One of the more interesting ways to study this possibility involved the subject's choice of wearing apparel. A textile company had subjects choose the heaviness of the clothing they would wear depending on receiving (or not receiving) a period of bright light in the late afternoon and early evening.The bright light resulted in the subjects picking heavier clothing, and they indeed produced more melatonin and had a deeper body temperature drop.

CHAPTER 4.

The Toronto Experiment

Ever since the early 1990s, scientists have been warning that using light at night increases the risk of cancer. Dr. Hahn, an epidemiologist at the National Institute of Environmental Health Sciences, found that blind women had only about half the incidence of breast cancer as women with normal vision. He suspected it was because blind women didn't experience melatonin suppression due to light exposure and that having more melatonin protected the women from breast cancer. Dr. Schoenhammer at Harvard, also an epidemiologist, examined breast cancer incidence and found that nurses who had worked nightshift for a long time (fifteen years) had a significantly higher incidence of breast cancer than nurses who did not work nightshift.

Meanwhile, a research group at the University of Toronto set out to demonstrate that nightshift workers did not need to be deprived of their melatonin. They studied a group of volunteers who maintained a normal schedule of sleeping during the night and measured the melatonin in their saliva every half hour during the night while they were in darkness. On a subsequent night, they took samples during the night while the volunteers worked a simulated nightshift under well-lighted conditions. After a few normal days, they worked another simulated nightshift under well-lighted conditions, except this time they wore goggles that blocked the blue light that causes melatonin suppression.

On the night they were in darkness, the volunteers produced a normal rise and fall of the melatonin in their saliva. (By the way, earlier experiments determined that the amount of melatonin in the saliva tracks its blood concentration very well.) On the night they worked the nightshift under well-lighted conditions, they produced almost no melatonin. On the night they worked the nightshift with goggles, they produced melatonin just as they had while in darkness.

During the night they worked the simulated nightshift wearing goggles, the subjects were asked to take a number of tests to indicate alertness, sleepiness, and manual skills. All the tests indicated they were not exhibiting outward signs of having melatonin present. Healthy, highly motivated young people can probably do an isolated nightshift and produce large amounts of melatonin without exhibiting drowsiness.

As a policy, having regular nightshift workers wear blue-blocking glasses to produce melatonin during the night while working is probably a mistake. The proper way to deal with nightshift work is to shift the circadian clock so that melatonin is flowing during the time the worker is sleeping. If the person is working 11:00 p.m. to 7:00 a.m. and sleeping from 9:00 a.m. to 5:00 p.m., putting on blue-blocking glass at 8:00 a.m. and sleeping in the dark from nine to five will eventually allow the melatonin to flow coincidently with the hours of sleep. Exposing the eyes to bright light on arising and during the remainder of the awake time will help avoid sleepiness.

Studies have shown that the majority of regular nightshift workers fail to do this. Social pressures to change to normal hours on weekends tend to mess up the schedule. Continually rotating shifts creates a really impossible situation as far as sleep is concerned and most likely creates a significant health threat.

Rotating shifts creates a situation closely analogous to jet lag problems. It is easier to prepare for eastward flight since it means advancing the circadian clock. Putting on blue-blocking glasses an hour earlier each night will shift the clock ahead. Going from L. A. to New York City is a three-hour difference so, for two nights, the glasses might go on an hour earlier and, on getting on the red-eye on the departure evening, the glasses would go on the third hour earlier. Using bright light on the morning of arrival should consolidate the time change. In planning for rotating shifts, moving the schedule as if going east would be desirable in terms of trying to keep melatonin flowing during the sleep time. There may be more compelling reasons to move the schedule in the other direction. Providing eight more hours to make the adjustment may be sufficient reason.

CHAPTER 5.

How People Study Sleep

Some of the most interesting studies of sleep have been done by Dr. Czeisler and his students at Harvard Medical School. His studies follow a well-worn path in that they make use of the "dim light onset of melatonin," DLMO, as a way of determining in a highly controlled way how the circadian clock is set.

For example, for three days the subjects follow a highly regulated routine of eight hours of sleep in darkness and sixteen hours of uniform light at either 200 lux or 0.5 lux. After a fourth set of eight hours of sleep in darkness, they are exposed to a period of forty hours of dim light during which the blood is sampled to measure the melatonin flow. For more than twenty-four hours there has been no visual cue or other signal to indicate the time of day, but still the body clock turns on the flow of melatonin at the expected time. The expected time is during the period the subjects had been in darkness during the previous three days. The flow started within a few minutes (+ or -) of the time they had been going into darkness and lasted well past the eight hours.

This longer flow of melatonin when in darkness or dim light is the factor we are missing when we use artificial light of moderate intensity up to the time we go to bed and again first thing on rising. There is a fairly large difference in melatonin production between different individuals. In this experiment, there is about a four-fold difference in the amount of melatonin produced between the subjects with the least and most melatonin. The purpose of the experiment I am describing is to determine whether the long-term prior exposure to different light levels has an effect on the suppression of melatonin caused by light.

After three more days made up of eight hours of sleep in darkness and sixteen hours of exposure to 200 lux, the melatonin flow was again monitored using the time when the subjects had been sleeping, but now the light was kept on at 200 lux. Two things happened. First the flow was delayed by several hours in most subjects and greatly reduced in all subjects but by different amounts. Average reduction was 71%.

The next experiment was to have three days made up of eight hours of sleep in darkness and sixteen hours of exposure to 0.5 lux (very dim light). At the end of the third day, instead of going into darkness and sleep, the subjects were exposed to six and a half hours of 200 lux of light. In this case the melatonin flow was delayed for the full six and a half hours for most subjects and suppressed considerably more than in the earlier case. The average reduction was 86%. Clearly a form of adaptation had occurred when the eyes had been exposed to 200 lux as described in the previous paragraph so that the suppression was less. It suggests very strongly that if you have been in darkness for a number of hours, it may not take much light to kill your melatonin. It strongly suggests that if you get up at night to use the bathroom, don't turn on the light.

This experiment fails to answer the question of whether long-term adaptation (three days) is required, or if only a shorter period of hours before the light exposure would be sufficient. It also provides little information on the practical question of what happens to the melatonin cycle in a typical home setting. It does, however, provide the warning that prior light exposure needs to be accounted for in any experiments designed to study melatonin suppression.

Perhaps what may be surprising to some people is the robust nature of the melatonin cycle. Without any clues from the surroundings, the cycle turns on with only the information from the internal clock. Studies have shown that when there is no light exposure to reset the internal clock that its natural day length is slightly more than twenty-four hours. This is why daily exposure to both light and darkness at a consistent hour are important for good sleep and good mood. It keeps the body in synch with the natural world.

Those who study sleep divide it into four or five stages depending on who is doing the dividing. The sleep stage everyone has heard about is rapid eye movement sleep, called REM sleep, which is also abbreviated that way. It is the stage where most dreaming occurs and during which muscles are paralyzed. It is surmised that this is a protective development so we can't act out our dreams and get hurt.

Study of brain waves from an EEG is one of the ways the different stages of sleep are identified. REM sleep is characterized by waves that are similar to those we produce when awake. The other stages of sleep feature waves that vary in frequency and amplitude.

Normal sleep is characterized by the body going through the different stages in a repetitive manner so that each cycle lasts about 1.5 hours or so. In a typical night there might be five cycles in which the duration of REM sleep gradually increases. In the time between the REM episodes, one goes through the deepest sleep, when it is difficult to wake a person. If a person is wakened during REM sleep he is likely to report having been dreaming. When a new customer for the blue-blocking glasses reports the results of trying them for a while, a frequent comment is how his dreams have become so vivid. He may also comment that he believes it is because he is sleeping more soundly. Whatever the explanation, it has become such a common comment it appears to be a real effect.

CHAPTER 6.

The Problems With Sleeping Pills

One of the compelling reasons to promote the drug-free method of improving sleep by controlling light in the hours before bedtime is the rapidly growing use of sleeping pills. I've seen the statement that 47 million subscriptions for sleeping pills were written in 2005, up some 20% from 2002. This is just in the United States. While sleeping pills obviously have their value, they also include risk. Unfortunately, many people who are taking sleeping pills are totally unaware of the unfortunate experiences that have resulted from not following the instructions that come with the pills. Even when following instructions, there can be serious side effects.

Ambien (Zolpidem), which has about 70% of the sleeping pill sales in the United States, is recommended for only brief usage of seven to fourteen days, but is most commonly available in thirty-tablet bottles. The manufacturer, Sanofi-Aventis, warns against combining Ambien with alcohol. This is probably the most common type of abuse. A man reported taking an Ambien after having a single alcoholic drink some time before and then proceeded, after a couple of hours, to take the remaining thirteen Ambien tablets. His daughter found him unconscious and called for help. Fortunately he survived but had no recollection of having taken the additional pills. He was not depressed or unhappy about anything. He could not understand why he had done what he did.

A distraught father whose daughter committed suicide after having taken Ambien has launched a website (www.randis-quest.info) with the intent of providing warning to others of the dangers. His daughter was not depressed; nevertheless, she shot herself on arising on the first night after having taken a sample of Ambien given to her by her doctor. She had also been taking Wellbrutin, so it's not completely clear if there may have been drug interactions.

To have a few problems is perhaps not surprising when you consider that 47 million prescriptions for sleeping pills were written in 2005, the majority for Ambien. According to an article from the New York *Times* written by Stephanie Saul, many states do not test for Ambien when a driver is charged with driving under the influence. In ten of the twenty-four states that do test for Ambien, it makes the top ten list. In Minnesota, where they do test for Ambien, they found 187 drivers over a period of five years whose blood contained Ambien. In Washington State they found Ambien in the blood of seventy-eight drivers in 2005, up from fifty-six in 2004.

In addition to the problems associated with combining sleeping pills and alcohol and the problem of driving when under their influence, there may be side effects when the sleeping pills are taken as directed. These include next-day sleepiness, amnesia, dizziness, hallucinations, delusions, altered thought patterns, increased appetite, decreased libido, depression, anxiety, impaired judgment, increased impulsivity and rebound insomnia when stopped. Hopefully some of the nine new ones that are in Phase II clinical trials and the seven that are in Phase III clinical trials will have fewer side effects.

A newly approved (July 2005) sleeping pill, ramelteon (Rozerem), is a chemical analog of melatonin and affects the melatonin receptors throughout the body much as melatonin does. Because it has FDA approval for treating insomnia, doctors can prescribe it. It appears to be nearly free of next-day problems and appears to be non-addictive.

In the United States melatonin is not a controlled substance and has never been tested or approved by the FDA. It is available without a prescription and is sold at most drug stores and health food stores.

The tricky thing about using it for treating insomnia is that the required dose when taking it orally, is highly variable from one person to the next. I've read that a very small dose of less than one milligram works better for insomnia than larger doses. The timing is also very important.

If taken at the wrong time of day, it can reset the internal clock. This may produce more severe insomnia. Because of the uncertainty surrounding taking melatonin by mouth, we don't recommend it unless blocking blue light in the evening does not work.

Another problem with sleeping pills is that the body becomes more tolerant of them after long-time use and they stop working. This is not a problem in using the glasses to promote the body's own melatonin production. It is a return to the natural conditions we experienced before the invention of electric lights.

CHAPTER 7.

Developing Lights That Don't Suppress Melatonin

If ordinary lights used at night are causing cancer, something needs to be done about it. Consider how many years elapsed after it was first suspected that smoking cigarettes caused lung cancer before there was agreement by the medical profession about the dangers. In retrospect it is hard to understand why this was the case. The medical profession does not use logic alone in making decisions. They rely almost entirely on the results of large clinical trials before taking any action. Fortunately individuals are not so limited. At the first suggestion that cigarettes caused lung cancer, thousands of people quit. They were glad years later that they had.

What's the analogy here? I don't think many people are going to give up electric lights. Fortunately the fact that it is only the blue component in light that causes melatonin suppression means we only need to block blue light. And we only need to do this at night.

Certainly one approach is to have lights that don't produce blue light. To this end the staff at the Lighting Innovations Institute at John Carroll University began measuring light sources that had coatings which absorbed blue light. Lights that are sold for use in studios where lithography is done use such lights as safe lights. Tubular fluorescent lamps are sold by the major manufacturers for this purpose.

Some bug lights with coatings that absorb some of the blue light were tested. Most only knocked out some of the blue light. A few knocked out almost all of it. Coatings were developed for compact fluorescent lamps that do a good job.

The problem with this approach is that to be effective, all of the lamps in the area where the person spends the evening need to be changed. Should hospitals install a dual lighting system, with one turned on only at night? Won't nurses working the nightshift get too sleepy? They should rather have their melatonin while they are off duty sleeping. What about the nurseries? There it does make sense. The nurses that are working in the nursery can experience white light to keep their melatonin suppressed when in the nurse's station next to the nursery. Rather than having the babies experience twenty-four hours of white light, turning on light that does not suppress melatonin for eight to twelve hours makes sense.

There are at least two reasons for protecting newborn infants from blue light. First there is the concern for retinal damage that has been discussed elsewhere and second there is recent evidence from studies with mice that show that when very young mice are exposed to continuous light they fail to develop a coherent circadian rhythm. It has been reported that infants kept in a neonatal unit for a long time have trouble sleeping normally when they go home.

Lighting for adult patients' rooms might well be equipped with yellow lights. Turning on such lights for an hour or two before normal lights-out and during the night when nurses must perform their procedures does make a lot of sense. For many hospitals, this might only require replacing a standard fluorescent lamp with a yellow one over each patient's bed. The neonatal units should consider having dual fixtures with white lights for daytime and lights without blue for nighttime. For children's rooms, it makes sense to have lights that do not suppress melatonin, especially for those children who are afraid of the dark. This way they can have enough light to chase away any scary shadows without keeping them awake for lack of melatonin.

CHAPTER 8.

Treating Jet Lag

While jet lag is not really an illness, it is analogous to delayed phase sleep disorder that is treated as an illness. It really depends on which direction you are traveling. If you are going east, it is analogous to delayed phase, but if you are going west, it is like advance phase sleep disorder. If you are traveling east, the clock says it is time to go to bed but you are still wide awake and going strong. If you go west, the problem is trying to stay awake when you are still supposed to be having fun.

To avoid jet lag takes some planning ahead. Studies have shown that it is possible to move your circadian clock ahead about one hour per day. You can do this by putting on blue-blocking glasses about an hour before your normal bedtime on the first day of preparation. The next evening, you put on the glasses two hours before your normal bedtime, and on the third evening of preparation, you put them on three hours before your normal bedtime. If you are departing the next day, you put on the glasses four hours before your normal bedtime while you are most likely on your way. If your destination is England, your circadian clock should be pretty well set to the new time. Getting plenty of light in the early morning will help reinforce the new time.

Going west requires using the glasses in the morning to delay your circadian rhythm. For a four-hour delay, you will need to put on the glasses for an hour after awakening on the fourth day preceding your trip. You will extend the time for an hour each day. Staying up, exposing your eyes to light for an hour longer each evening, will also help. Shifting your eating time to a later hour will also help.

CHAPTER 9.

The Sleepy Student Problem

One of the biggest problems faced by school boards is how to fit everything into a school day. It isn't just the academic activities, but all of the extra things that go on in a modern high school.Transportation is a major problem, with most children being bussed to school. Getting them there is a different problem from taking them home because of the myriad of after-school activities.There are not only all the continually changing sports programs but also marching band practice, school plays, and on and on.To fit this all into a reasonable schedule requires getting things started early, which ends up with school starting mighty early.This may be okay for younger children because parents are able to get them to bed early, but for high school age children, it presents a serious challenge. Many high school students are only half awake during the early classes. Researchers have measured melatonin levels in high school students during early classes and found that many still have high levels in their blood.

A number of school districts have revised their starting time to take this into account, but not without much effort and discussion. If the high school students would simply go to bed earlier it would solve the problem, but apparently this is an impossible requirement.

Fortunately there is an answer to the problem that doesn't require changing the starting time. If the students simply put on the blue- blocking glasses at a reasonable hour, their melatonin cycle will end before school starts and they can stay up as late as they want. Since the glasses will probably make them feel drowsy, they may decide to go to bed a bit earlier, which will pay dividends in their ability to learn the following day.

CHAPTER 10.

Sleep and Mental Illness

It has been observed for many years that people with some forms of mental illness do not sleep well. Only very recently have people been thinking about this the other way around. Perhaps they become mentally ill because they don't sleep well. Bipolar disorder used to be called manic depressive illness. It is characterized by people who go from one extreme to the other. For a while they are on the top of the world and feeling just great and then they plunge into the depths of depression. Some early studies found that when people went into depression it was usually after sleeping rather than at the end of a period of being awake. The manic mood was more likely to begin toward the middle or end of a period of being awake. Researchers tried things like sleep deprivation to get people out of depression since it was thought that sleep was causing depression.

One of the bodily parameters that is easy to measure is core body temperature. In general, it varies the opposite way as the concentration of the melatonin in the blood. It is highest during the day when melatonin is absent and drops to a minimum when melatonin concentration is at a maximum. In more recent studies, it has been plotted against time for patients with rapid cycling bipolar disorder. The results showed that it cycled up and down but not in synchronization with the twenty-four-hour clock. It was free running, going in and out of phase with the patient's schedule of waking and sleeping. The patient's mood was cycling up and down, but in a very irregular fashion.

Now, rather than trying sleep deprivation, a novel approach was tried, known as "darkness therapy." The patient was placed in a darkened room for fourteen hours a day, not required to sleep, but simply to be in the darkness from about 6 p.m. to 8 a.m. After just a few days, the patient's mood became stable and the body temperature cycle was locked in with the twenty-four-hour clock. The period of darkness was decreased to twelve hours and the mood continued to be stable. A similar approach was tried with sixteen rapid cycling bipolar patients in Italy with similar results for new patients without a long history of bipolar disorder.

These studies strongly support the notion that bipolar disorder is somehow associated with abnormal functioning of the circadian clock. This fits with the early observations that the manic phase could be triggered by erratic behavior involving staying up until the small hours of the morning. Exposing the eyes to light during the night could have a disruptive effect on the circadian clock. Whatever the explanation of how the clock gets out of order, darkness therapy has been demonstrated as a way to get it back to normal for some patients.

With the present theory of melatonin suppression by blue light, it is possible to produce "virtual darkness" by simply putting on blue- blocking glasses. This makes getting fourteen hours of darkness very easy. Putting on the glasses at 6 p.m., going to bed at midnight in real darkness, and getting up at 8 a.m. is all very simple, easy, and not disruptive of normal evening activities. Hopefully experience will show this as another tool to deal with a very difficult condition.

CHAPTER 11.

A Safer Method of Treating Seasonal Affective Disorder (SAD)

SAD is experienced by a large fraction of the population, especially women. It is a mild to severe depression that occurs every year in the winter season, particularly in the higher latitudes where the hours of darkness reach high values. Combining this with cold temperatures and gray skies is enough to make anyone feel at least a bit depressed. A number of the doctors who started out trying to prove the condition was strictly psychological ended up believing it has a physiological basis. Many have come to believe it is the result of melatonin continuing to exist in the blood well past the time it should be gone. One piece of evidence for this is the success obtained using light boxes to treat SAD.

While not in the same class of mental illness as bipolar disorder, the condition called seasonally affective disorder, or SAD, is still serious when viewed from the perspective of those who suffer from it. It is quite a common condition, especially at higher latitudes where winter nights are very long and sunlight is at a premium. The standard treatment has been to use light therapy early in the morning. Recently the very high brightness white light boxes that usually use fluorescent lamps have been replaced with lower brightness blue LED illuminators. This is based on the work of Brainard and Skene on the action spectrum for melatonin suppression. The success achieved with the blue LED sources is evidence for the hypothesis that SAD is the result of having melatonin in the bloodstream in the morning, which makes the subjects feel tired and depressed. Exposing the eyes to the light causes the pineal gland to stop making melatonin, and after a half hour or so the kidneys remove the melatonin from the blood and people feel better.

This method of treating SAD is not without some risk. Blue light is known to cause damage to the retina, which ultimately may result in macular degeneration and partial blindness in some individuals. The risk is small but not zero. Because this process is believed to be photochemical in nature rather than thermal, there is no completely safe level. In photochemical reactions, each photon is capable of breaking a chemical bond and doing its damage. In thermal damage, it requires many photons arriving at a certain rate to raise the temperature of the cells enough to cause permanent damage. The blue light damage is thus dependent on how many of the blue photons have arrived at the retina over a long period of time.

A new treatment for SAD is completely free from the retinal hazard of blue light. It depends on advancing the melatonin cycle so that it finishes before the individual awakens. This is made possible by donning blue-blocking glasses in the early evening. After doing this regularly for several consecutive days, the melatonin cycle will be advanced in time. Many studies have shown that the melatonin cycle will not last more than nine or ten hours even when no light is present to suppress it, e.g. as in blind people.

If the glasses are put on regularly at 9 p.m., the cycle will start by no later than 10 p.m. and finish no later than 8 a.m. If this is not early enough, the glasses may be put on at 8 p.m. to allow the cycle to finish by 7 a.m. Since the glasses only block the blue light, the other colors of light are available for reading, working on a computer or watching television. This method of treating SAD is perfectly safe and has the additional advantage that people afflicted with SAD don't have to stop what they are doing and sit in front of a light box for half an hour.

Not all SAD is necessarily due to the presence of melatonin in the blood. Some may be purely psychological, and exposing the eyes to light my help that condition. It is likely that that condition may be treated more successfully by simply providing bright and cheerful surroundings in the morning without the need to sit in front of a light box.

CHAPTER 12.

Postpartum Depression

The depression following child birth has sometimes been called the "baby blues." Most new mothers suffer from it to some extent. This is a period of rapid change in hormone balance, and it usually passes in a week or two. Approximately 10–15% of new mothers suffer from a more prolonged and deeper feeling of sadness to the point of seeking some kind of help. This is called postpartum depression (ppd). It is usually treated with an anti-depressant drug and frequently by providing support such as group therapy. A few women develop psychosis following the birth of a baby that may include delusions and mania as well as depression. Hospitalization may be required to treat these women.

In the past few years, a number of popular books have exposed the degree to which postpartum depression may destroy not only the happiness of the mother but also that of the father and child. Several celebrities have suffered from ppd and have described their experiences. Actress Brooke Shields had a great deal of trouble becoming pregnant, had a miscarriage, finally became pregnant again, had a horrible delivery, and went into a deep depression over a long time. She finally recovered with the help of medicine and therapy. Her book *Down Came the Rain* is a moving account of her ordeal.

In accounts of ppd, the common thread running through most of them is insomnia, the inability to get restful sleep even though exhausted. I've heard the expression "too tired to sleep" and always thought it was similar to the incorrect expression "too cold to snow." It's never too cold to snow. With our knowledge of melatonin and circadian disruption, it is now possible to understand being "too tired to sleep." It's not the exhaustion that is the problem. It may be the lack of melatonin or its arrival at the wrong time.

There is considerable evidence that depression is associated with disruption of the circadian cycle or, perhaps more correctly, that disrupting the circadian rhythm may result in depression.

When a baby is born, the normal sleep routine of the mother is interrupted frequently by the needs of the baby. When she gets up to change and feed the baby, she normally does this in a lighted room where the light may cause a reduction in the flow of melatonin. If this happens several times a night, the result may be both a reduction in the amount of melatonin produced and a disruption of her circadian cycle. This may mean that the following night her melatonin flow may not begin at the usual time, and although she may be very tired, she may not be able to fall asleep quickly. As this sequence continues, it may lead to a deep depression.

It is not completely understood why some women suffer from ppd and why most do not. There are clearly certain indicators that a woman may have a problem. Some women experience some signs of mental instability at puberty in association with their periods, and when becoming pregnant. If this is the case, there is a high probability they will also suffer ppd. This information supports the view that hormonal changes in women's bodies are at the root of ppd. Use of a series of ten questions called the EDSD as soon as seven days after delivery has been shown to quite accurately predict if the woman will have a problem with ppd. Other similar tests have been developed to help screen those women who will need help.

This situation may be avoided, or at least minimized, by avoiding light that contains the blue part of the spectrum. Using products that prevent blue light from entering the eye may offer some help. By a very simple change in lifestyle the mother may avoid having her melatonin flow interrupted. When she needs to take care of her baby, all that is necessary is for her to put on glasses that block the melatonin- suppressing light before she turns on any light. Alternatively, the rooms in which she takes care of her baby may be lighted with lamps with filters that block the melatonin-suppressing light. Using such lights may also be beneficial to the baby by not suppressing his/her melatonin.

If the new mother is breastfeeding her baby, she may also maximize her own melatonin and the amount in her breast milk by putting on blue-blocking glasses or turning on lamps with filters so that her melatonin flow will begin a few hours earlier than normal. Studies have shown that nine to ten hours of melatonin flow are possible. Newborn babies produce little melatonin on their own. Melatonin in the mother's breast milk may be responsible for the commonly held impression that breast-fed babies sleep better. This is not simply an impression but was borne out of studies in which melatonin metabolite was measured in the urine of breastfed babies. It was largely missing in the urine of bottle-fed babies.

The vicious cycle of the mother's lack of melatonin in her milk and the baby not sleeping well is documented in a number of studies. This is where providing help so the mother can get some solid sleep can pay dividends in breaking the vicious cycle. There is one study that supports the notion that keeping the mother's circadian cycle operating normally—that is, she produces melatonin during the night—will help her breastfed baby develop a circadian cycle that agrees with hers. Having a baby on a schedule like the mother's is of tremendous value to both.

Many men, about 10% of new fathers, also suffer depression following the birth of a baby, especially if the mother is suffering from ppd. While depression is the most common manifestation, anxiety is frequently also present. Fathers frequently encounter the same problem of exposing their eyes to light during the night when helping with the baby, particularly if the mother is incapacitated with ppd. The fact that almost as many men suffer from ppd as women is very strong evidence that the problem is not primarily due to disruption of hormones. This speaks very strongly in support of the idea that exposure of the eyes to light with subsequent disruption of the circadian cycle and sleep deprivation are more likely the cause of the depression.

There is a great deal of evidence that ppd is not only damaging to the mother and father, but also to the baby in the form of poor sleep and emotional neglect. We tend to think of ppd as being a short-term problem, but many women suffer for many months and sometimes years. The lack of bonding between the mother and the child described in many accounts of ppd is perhaps the saddest result which can have long-term consequences. One study of depressed mother-child pairs when the baby was about three months old showed there was less vocal and visual communication, less corporeal interactions, and less smiling than in a control group in which there was no depression.

One study of slightly older children found that the mother's current depressive symptoms have stronger influence than earlier depressive symptoms, with mothers not initiating recommended age-appropriate safety and child development practices and also using harsh discipline practices for toddlers. The findings, however, also suggest that for parenting practices that are likely to be established early in the life of the child, it may be reasonable that mothers with early depressive symptoms may continue to affect use of those practices

One study with four-month-old children of depressed mothers and non-depressed fathers found that the infants did not respond to the mother's voice or to that of other non-depressed women but did respond to the father's voice. This would be devastating to a mother.

There are many studies attesting to the fact that postpartum depression is a problem found in technically advanced countries. Data from countries without electric lighting would be very helpful in determining whether electric lighting does play a large role in developing ppd. The much lower rate of cancer in primitive societies is well documented, with melatonin, and its suppression by light, being thought to provide the link.

For those who have already succumbed to postpartum depression, recovery will be accelerated by avoiding ordinary light at night. Installing special nursery lights and using the glasses regularly will help the sufferer get back on track. Exposing the eyes to ordinary light at more or less the same time every morning will also help reset the circadian clock so that it agrees with the clock on the wall. Getting melatonin to flow during the night when it should flow will be a big help.

CHAPTER 13.

The Shift Work Dilemma

A higher risk of illness for people working nightshift has not been shown in most epidemiological studies. The higher risk seems to occur for those who work rotating or swing shifts or occasionally work nightshifts. This makes sense. Those who normally work the second or third shift have an opportunity to adjust their circadian rhythms so that they produce melatonin during the hours they sleep and do not produce it during their working hours. On the other hand, those who are constantly changing from one shift to another probably don't get sufficiently adjusted to the new shift before they are shifted to the next one.

Advancing the circadian rhythm (like traveling in the eastward direction) seems to be easier than the reverse. This would suggest that the rotating shift should rotate in that way. That is, work two weeks third shift, two weeks second shift, and two weeks first shift, etc. This makes for short weekends and may not be popular with workers. It is much more attractive for a first shift worker on Friday to not have to report until second shift on Monday.

Using light in the evening to help these workers stay up later on Friday, Saturday, and Sunday evening may be of advantage, and possibly wearing glasses in the morning on Saturday, Sunday, and Monday morning may help move the clock to a later time. It would probably be most natural to plan to sleep midnight to 8 a.m. when working second shift.

Moving to third shift is difficult. Working second shift Friday evening would require staying up for a couple of hours, say until 2 a.m. on

Saturday morning and until 4 a.m. on Sunday morning and then begin third shift at midnight Sunday night (Monday morning).

For those who regularly work at night and sleep during the day, the goal is to try to make the daytime sleeping as much like nighttime sleeping as possible. This means blackout shades for the windows and earplugs to reduce the noise. Use of a white noise generator is helpful in blocking out distracting sounds. As regular a schedule as possible is recommended. Wearing glasses that block blue light for an hour or two before going to bed is recommended to help in falling asleep quickly. If it becomes necessary to get up during your sleep period, avoid exposing the eyes to light, since it may kill melatonin production and tends to reset your circadian clock. Once you have succeeded in convincing your body that night is day, you need to keep reinforcing that setting by keeping on a regular schedule, even on weekends, as much as possible.

Dr. Eastman and her colleagues at Rush Hospital in Chicago have studied the problems of sleep for people working nightshift. Reading their many papers on www.Pubmed.gov may be of value to those who work rotating shifts. They suggest that complete adjustment of the circadian clock to provide for melatonin flow coincident with sleep is not the best goal since it leaves these workers misaligned for doing things during the day on their days off. In one of their papers they propose a compromise solution in which the circadian rhythm is delayed only enough that the core body temperature minimum occurs during the early part of the morning sleep schedule (8:30 a.m-3:30 p.m.). This allows for weekend activities beginning in late morning or at noon, without extreme fatigue. They can accomplish the phase shifting by five 15-minute exposures to bright light (3500 lux) during the night shift (11:00 p.m.- 7:00 a.m.) and wearing blue-blocking glasses on the way home after the nightshift.

CHAPTER 14.

Sunlight and the Human Body

Most people crave the light of the sun. Every year we spend millions of dollars traveling to places where we can soak up those wonderful rays. We love to lie in the sun. We love to get a tan. There is a steady migration to the "sunshine states."

In recent years, there have been many warnings by the medical profession of the dangers posed by exposure to sunlight. The public has become so concerned about this that now the doctors are warning about not getting enough sunlight.

Light at wavelengths toward the blue-violet end of the visible spectrum and beyond in the ultraviolet is essentially different from longer wavelength light. The difference is that each photon has sufficient energy to cause chemical reactions in the form of breaking chemical bonds between atoms that make up molecules. X-rays and cosmic rays and some rays from nuclear reactions have this kind of effect on organic molecules. These kinds of effects are referred to as photochemical reactions.

Longer wavelength light in the red and near infrared part of the spectrum does not have sufficient energy in each photon to do this. It may, however, have enough energy to lift an electron out of its normal orbit and make it available to another atom. These kinds of photoelectric effects can also result in chemical change. Photosynthesis of green plants is the main way we capture energy from the sun and make both food and fuel and renew the oxygen in our atmosphere. In contrast, the longer wavelength electromagnetic energy is called infrared and it produces its effects primarily by raising the temperature of materials that absorb it.

The basis for concern about exposure to the ultraviolet rays in sunshine is primarily about melanoma, a very deadly skin cancer. The precise manner in which sunlight causes melanoma is not understood. It seems to be a cumulative effect over a long time. Children exposed to a lot of sunlight are more prone to develop melanoma in later life. It is thought to be related to damage in the DNA of the cells. There is concern that the reduction in the ozone layer that allows more UV to reach the surface of the earth will result in an increase in melanoma. Antioxidants which can destroy cells with damaged DNA help with recovery from sun damage. Melatonin is a powerful antioxidant. It is logical to expect that increasing the time when melatonin is present in the body will help reduce the risk of melanoma as well as other types of cancer.

The best defense against melanoma is keeping a watchful eye on any moles or other skin imperfections for any sign of change in appearance. It's not just black or dark brown moles that may become a problem. They can be any color or multicolored. They can appear on any part of the body but more commonly on parts that may be exposed to the sun. Because melanoma has a strong tendency to spread to other parts of the body, it is very important to have a suspicious lesion surgically removed as quickly as possible.

Sunburn is another, but less serious, type of damage to the skin produced by ultraviolet light. The fact that the effect is delayed makes relying on common sense more difficult. Damage is done before it is noticed. Since sunscreen lotions are in common usage, bad sunburns are much less common.

Blue light damage to the eye has been studied extensively. Inflammation of the retina is called retinitis. It is perhaps surprising that not more cases of retinitis occur from people just changing light bulbs or trying to read the wattage of operating lamps. The danger from clear ordinary incandescent light bulbs and halogen light bulbs is very much greater. Just a few seconds of exposure can cause serious eye damage since the lens of the eye focuses an image of the filament on the retina. Just glancing at a clear bulb can cause prolonged after images. If an after image lasts for more than thirty seconds, it suggests borderline damage may have been done. Fortunately we tend to squint or close our eyes when they are hit with a bright light. Damage to the eye is very common at the time of an eclipse. People should never try to get even a glimpse of the sun without protection.

There is another concern for eye damage by blue light associated with macular degeneration. The macula of the retina is the area where blood vessels enter the retina and spread out over the whole surface. Macular degeneration involves leakage of blood from these vessels that obscures the central portion of the retina where vision is most acute, causing partial blindness.

While the evidence that blue light causes macular degeneration is not very strong, those who study it suggest it is wise to be on the safe side and avoid unnecessary exposure by wearing eyewear that blocks blue light. This is particularly true for fair people with blue eyes. Sunglasses that are available as "blue-blockers" are recommended. They not only block the blue light but enough of other wavelengths to make being outside much more comfortable. These glasses are not suitable for use indoors at night since they are much too dark.

Wearing these sunglasses outside at all times is probably not a good idea either, especially in the morning. To keep the circadian clock set to the desired time, exposure to light in the early morning seems to be required. A number of authors suggest fifteen minutes is adequate. A number also suggest outdoor light is most effective. More than likely, eating breakfast in a bright, cheerful kitchen may do the job. The blue LED light boxes are a possible source of damage to the eyes and are not recommended in this book.

CHAPTER 15.

Why Don't We Have Any Competition?

Just because it's logical doesn't mean it's right. Call it human nature, but people are extremely skeptical that something as simple as putting on a pair of glasses is going to change anything. And in a sense they are right. For people who do not have a sleeping problem, wearing glasses for a few hours before bedtime wouldn't appear to have much effect. The main effect we have observed in clinical trials of people without sleep problems has been a more regular pattern of sleeping in terms of number of hours each night and quality of sleep. Some people report falling asleep more quickly. The long-term benefits of having melatonin present for a longer time are not easily noticed. These are mostly the absence of health problems.

Using just "melatonin" as the search word in www.Pubmed.gov results in 13,360 abstracts of papers documenting the many ways melatonin is of benefit. During just the first half of 2007, 780 papers were published about the benefits of melatonin. These range from improving the health of gum tissue to reducing the toxic effects of cadmium (similar to mercury) to avoiding glaucoma and regression of endometriosis. There is increasing confidence that marketing products that block blue light will gradually become a significant business. About the time it does is when we discover a host of competitors. Some companies have a policy of normally being second with new products. Let the pioneer spend all the money figuring it out.

CHAPTER 16.

How This Journey Began

For a number of years I had been working on the application of the rapidly improving Light Emitting Diodes (LEDs) to a variety of lighting tasks, such as providing exterior lighting of a concept car for Mitsubishi and running lights for ships. I was approached by a friend who wanted us to design an LED light for treating Seasonal Affective Disorder (SAD) using blue LEDs. Such light boxes were already available, but used many LEDs and were expensive. His idea was to use just one of the higher power LEDs and make a very compact, inexpensive device. Working on that project got me interested in the whole subject of how light might impact human health.

Until I began learning more, I had believed that SAD was simply the psychological effect of dark winter mornings which made a few neurotic women feel depressed and that turning on some bright lights brightened their spirits. Apparently I was not alone in this belief. Many doctors simply dismissed this condition as "all in your head." It wasn't until I had learned the whole story about blue light and melatonin that I came to believe SAD was a real condition caused by residual melatonin in the blood that could be relieved with blue light to stop the flow and kidney action to eliminate it from the blood.

Vilnis Kubulins and I had worked on the LED blue light for treating SAD. Vilnis is a Research Associate who had worked with Dr. Carome for more than ten years after getting a master's degree in physics at JCU. The other active member of Lighting Innovations was Dr. Edward Carome, a retired physics professor with whom I had worked on several contracts for the Federal Aviation Administration. He was closely following that development since he was working on similar LED projects for Siemens Airfield Solutions. They were sponsoring some of our research on replacing incandescent air field lighting with LEDs. He was working on a runway stop light at the time.

As I continued looking at the effect of light on the body, it wasn't long before I came across the studies of nurses who worked nightshifts and their increased incidence of breast cancer. That was quite a shock for someone who had spent an entire career developing better and brighter light bulbs. Was I an unwitting accomplice in the suffering and death of thousands of women? This was the real beginning of what has gradually become a mission to alert people to the danger and provide a means of avoiding it.

The first thing we thought should be done was to make light bulbs that did not produce the offending blue light. That turned out to be easy in one sense but elusive in another. We started out by testing the emission from a number of light bulbs on the market as decorative lamps or as "bug lights." Some were good and some were not, but we found a few that we were confident were safe. We also found some fluorescent lamps, both tubular and compact, that met our criteria of almost no light at wavelengths less than 530nm. The only problem was we could not find any higher wattage lamps with the right filtering action. We set out to get some coated ourselves using pigment that appeared perfect. After working for a couple of years on it, we still do not have a coating for either compact fluorescent or incandescent lamps of higher light output that lasts for the life of the lamp. It seems like such a simple problem, but so far the solution eludes us.

The more we thought about it, the more obvious it became that safe light bulbs were not the optimum answer for most people. To be effective, it required that one stay in a room equipped with the special lamps or to put them all over the house. A more practical idea was to block the blue light at the eyes instead of at the source. Again, this did not require actual development, but rather simply required searching and finding existing products we could offer to the public as safe from the damaging blue light.

There are many "blue-blocking" glasses sold as sunglasses. Rather than only blocking all the light shorter than 530nm, they also block some of the light at longer wavelengths. This is not what we want. We want to block all the light at shorter wavelengths but as little as possible of the remaining spectrum since we want to be able to carry on normal evening activities. We have been able to locate several sources of glasses that do this. We are still searching for some with a bit more style than the ones we have located so far.

Dr. Carome decided to try the glasses himself. He had had sleeping problems for many years and wondered if the glasses might help him. They seemed to work the first night he tried them. For a number of days he continued to try them and they continued to work. He was afraid to say anything to Vilnis or to me. He had enough experience to know that sometimes an experiment will seem to work beautifully and then when you try to repeat it, it fails to work at all.

But the glasses continued to work for him. His sleep was completely changed. Instead of waiting a long time to fall asleep, he fell asleep quickly, and instead of waking up many times during the night, he only had to get up once or twice and then fell asleep quickly.

We decided to initially offer them for sale on a website and, after some looking, picked a website designer. After she had it up and running in the summer of 2005, we put out a press release with the naïve thought that someone would notice. I sent a copy to Monica Robbins, health anchor at the local NBC outlet in Cleveland. We were very excited. She came out to the university with a cameraman and taped a ten-minute interview and took shots of some of our light bulbs and glasses.

We made ten seconds of our interview and eight seconds of our light bulbs on the 6 o'clock news and how this might help avoid skin cancer.

To her credit, Monica continues to express interest in our work and did put something on their website about avoiding postpartum depression when we began exploring that use.

Our business plan was equally naïve. It was to advertise our glasses locally to start with, and as sales picked up, to advertise them more broadly until we were running ads in the *New York Times* and selling thousand of glasses a day. The initial advertising was for a one-inch by two-inch ad in the *Chagrin Valley Times* (local paper for Chagrin Falls, Ohio) that comes out weekly. It cost $80 per week and we ran for three weeks. Not one sale resulted from these ads. They even ran a nice story about how the glasses were developed by scientists at John Carroll University and that many people found that by wearing them a few hours before bedtime they fell asleep more quickly and slept more soundly. The local business news *Crain's Cleveland Business* ran a nice story and picture about us and we did get a few sales from that story.

One of the big surprises was how deeply disinterested the cancer publications were in our efforts. We thought *Mamm* magazine, which is especially for women with breast cancer, would find our efforts of at least a little interest. No way! We tried to run an ad in *Coping* magazine that deals with cancer survivors, but they forced us to water down the ad so all we were saying is people might make more melatonin by wearing our glasses with no word about how that might reduce the risk of cancer.

We tried to get the *Cleveland Plain Dealer* to do an article about our efforts, but they were actually hostile and bragged about not being taken in by "those charlatans." Since improving sleep was much less controversial, we decided to put our efforts into promoting it and putting cancer in the background. We approached the head of alternative medicine at the Cleveland Clinic and gave her a few pair of glasses to try. She tried them on three long-term insomnia patients and reported back that she was in awe since all three were now "sleeping like babies." She continues to send patients to our website.

One of the sleep doctors we contacted fairly early on was Dr. Bert Briones, head of the sleep clinic at St. Vincent Charity Hospital. She expressed immediate interest and we provided her with a number of glasses that she tried with some of her patients. She continues to gather information and has observed mixed results. Clearly, if patients do not make much melatonin, they will not benefit from not suppressing what isn't there. If they are not exposing their eyes to enough light to suppress melatonin, there is nothing for the glasses to block.

We made presentations to other sleep specialists but soon came to realize that most of them were not all that interested in simple insomnia, but were more interested in doing the overnight sleep studies to identify sleep apnea and other more serious conditions for which they can do expensive tests and provide expensive equipment. I think they probably routinely prescribe Ambien or Lunesta for simple insomnia. They might only suggest our glasses if all else fails.

During the course of the first two years of our efforts, I composed six press releases that are reproduced here. They generated some interest and sales, but the effects were short lived.

New Glasses Prevent Jet Lag: No pills Required

University Heights, Ohio. January 29, 2006. University scientists have announced a new method to avoid jet lag. Many travelers have experimented with the hormone melatonin with limited success. The new method is more reliable because it uses the body's own melatonin. It's been known for many years that light striking the eye causes the pineal gland to stop making melatonin. Recently it has been discovered it is the blue component in white light that causes the suppression. New eyeglasses that block the blue light can allow travel to a distant place without the disruptive effects of jet lag. These glasses are available on the web at www.lowbluelights.com. The glasses have been checked with a spectrometer to be sure they block the light that causes melatonin suppression. This is a development from the Lighting Innovations Institute at John Carroll University in Cleveland, OH.

The traveler should begin adjusting his circadian clock to the new time zone a few days before departure. He can do this without actually having to adjust his daily pattern of living. For traveling east, he should put on the glasses an hour before normal bedtime the first night, two hours before bedtime the second night, etc. This gradually moves his circadian clock forward in time by starting melatonin flow at an earlier hour. By the time he leaves, his internal clock is running on the new time zone. Actually going to bed an hour earlier the night before departure will help make the change. After arrival he may find it beneficial to try exposure to bright lights first thing in the morning to cut off melatonin production. One theory is that there are two circadian clocks, one that turns on melatonin (in the absence of blue light) and a second that turns it off. The lights in the morning will reset the second circadian clock.

For traveling west, the traveler should start a few days before departure by putting on the glasses for an hour when he arises on the first day, for two hours the second, etc. This will push the circadian clock backward in time by allowing melatonin to flow past normal wake-up time. This may have the effect of making the traveler feel sleepy, so caution is required in using this method. On arrival he may want to have bright light available in the evening to prevent melatonin from starting to flow before he is ready to go to bed.

For traveling both east and west, a good general rule is to start in advance of departure one day for each time zone you are crossing. For a twelve-hour difference, the technique to use should depend on whether you are traveling east or west. Because melatonin is such a powerful hormone, it is not recommended taking it as a food supplement.

This application of the glasses is part of a more general effort to maximize the benefits of melatonin being carried out at John Carroll

University. Using light to control the body's melatonin offers a way to treat sleep problems. Making it available for longer times to fight cancer by wearing glasses in the evening is under ongoing study.

Trouble Sleeping? Colored Glasses Cure Insomnia.

Summary: The blue rays from artificial light stop production of melatonin, the sleep hormone. The cure is wearing glasses that block the damaging rays for a few hours before bedtime. Lots of melatonin becomes available by bedtime, so sleep comes quickly.

University Heights, OH, Mar. 22, 2006. Half of Americans claim they don't sleep well. Artificial light from lamps, TV, or computer screens in use in the hours before bedtime may be the major source of the sleep problem. It is well known that exposing the eyes to light prevents the pineal gland from making melatonin, the sleep hormone. Nerve fibers run from the eyes to the pineal gland and control when it produces melatonin and other hormones. It has only been known for several years that not all colors of light cause the suppression of melatonin. It is the light at the blue end of the visible spectrum that prevents melatonin production. This means that light bulbs can be made that do not eliminate melatonin secretion by coating them with filters that remove the blue rays that interfere with sleep. TV and computer screens may also be fitted with filters that remove the blue light that is creating sleep problems. An even more practical way to avoid the sleep problem is to wear glasses for a few hours before bedtime that block the blue rays. This permits reading, watching television, or working on a computer, without creating problems in going to sleep.

A clinical trial of glasses that block the blue light was carried out at the University of Toronto in which the subjects wearing the glasses continued making melatonin even though they were exposed to bright light. The same subjects without glasses on a different night failed to produce melatonin when exposed to the same lights. In preliminary experiments, subjects who have worn the glasses starting a few hours before their regular bedtime report falling asleep more quickly, sleeping more soundly, and feeling more rested in the morning. Some report a significant change in their sleep the first night they try the glasses that block the blue light.

Three physicists working in the Lighting Innovations Institute at John Carroll University in Cleveland came up with the idea of blocking the blue light to help people sleep better. They developed the light bulbs and glasses that avoid the problem of melatonin suppression. They formed a spin-off company, Photonic Developments, to market these products on the internet. The website is www.sleeplamps.com.

If you encounter any technical problems with ordering from the website, please call Dr. Hansler or send an email from the "contact" page. The website also contains many abstracts of scientific studies regarding sleep and melatonin along with popular articles on sleep and sleep problems. We would appreciate feedback about your experience with these exciting new products.

Contact person:
Dr. Richard L. Hansler
216 397 1657

Discovery Solves Problem of Early Starting Time of High Schools

Wearing blue-blocking eyeglasses a few hours before bedtime resets the internal clocks to an earlier hour.

A novel way to advance the circadian cycle has been proposed as a way to solve the problem associated with the early starting times of middle and high schools. It has been recognized for some time that teen age students do not really wake up until well past the time they physically arrive at school. Researchers at Brown University have found that the students' blood contains large amounts of the sleep hormone melatonin. Researchers at the Lighting Innovations Institute of John Carroll University are seeking funding to carry out a study to find out if their method of advancing the melatonin cycle will help.

It is well known that exposing the eyes to light during the evening delays the start of the flow of melatonin until after the person has gone into the darkness of the bedroom. Because the students like to stay up late working on their computers or watching television, their melatonin cycle is delayed. This means that in the morning, the cycle doesn't end until well after they are in school.

Five years ago it was discovered that not all light causes suppression of melatonin, only blue light. This means that wearing glasses that block blue light is the same as being in darkness as far as melatonin production is concerned. Putting on blue-blocking glasses at 9:00 p.m. will move the circadian cycle forward in time so that the melatonin flow is over before the student gets to school. A study at Harvard has found that blind people (who are in continual darkness) and normal sighted people, who are kept in darkness, make melatonin for 9-10 hours. If melatonin flow starts at 9:30 P.M. it will be over by 7:30 a.m..

The blue-blocking glasses have been tested as a means to help people with sleeping problems. Putting on the glasses a few hours before bedtime allows melatonin to be present at the time people go to bed. This avoids the delay in falling asleep experienced by many people. Using the glasses also has been reported to help people sleep more soundly. A double blind clinical trail of the amber glasses has shown a significant improvement in the quality of sleep and reduction of times awakening during the night when compared with placebo glasses that are light yellow and do not block the melatonin suppressing rays.

Wearing the glasses in the late evening results in getting close to the conditions of light and dark experienced before the invention of artificial lighting. Glasses that block the damaging blue light are available at a website of a spin-off company formed by the John Carroll researchers, www.lowbluelights.com. Filters for TV and computer screens as well as safe light bulbs are also available.

The John Carroll University researchers are seeking funding to test the glasses on high schools students to see if moving their circadian cycle forward in time will result in better academic performance in early morning classes.

Contact: Richard L. Hansler, Ph.D.
216 397 1657

Special Nursery Lights Help to Avoid Postpartum Depression

University scientists have developed special light bulbs for the nursery that don't give off the blue rays that cause melatonin suppression. They allow mothers to keep making melatonin when they get up at night to care for their babies. This prevents disrupting their circadian cycle. Many studies show that disruption of the circadian cycle can lead to depression.

University Heights, OH, Dec. 15, 2006 PRWebb: A light bulb specially designed for use in nurseries has been announced by physicists at John Carroll University. It features lack of the blue light rays known to cause suppression of melatonin, a hormone that promotes sleep. Lack of sleep and disruption of the circadian rhythm has been linked to depression. The new light bulb will help new mothers avoid post-partum depression.

It is estimated that 10–15 percent of births result in postpartum depression sufficiently serious to require treatment. It is generally accepted that rapidly changing hormone patterns are responsible. There is another factor that has been largely overlooked up until now: namely, the use of ordinary light during the night. Melatonin is produced by the pineal gland, but only when the eyes are in darkness. Normally the flow starts at night, a short time after going into a darkened bedroom, and gradually increases to a maximum about half-way through the night.

When a new mother gets up at night to take care of her baby and turns on an ordinary light, her pineal gland may stop making melatonin. When she goes back to bed she may have a hard time going back to sleep. If this happens several times a night, she may make little melatonin. If this happens every night for a number of nights in a row, it may totally disrupt her circadian cycle. This may lead to depression.

In 2001 it was discovered that not all light suppresses melatonin, only the blue rays. Experiments at the University of Toronto demonstrated that by blocking the blue rays, the pineal gland can continue making melatonin. Glasses that block blue light and light bulbs with filters to remove the blue light have been developed at John Carroll University in Cleveland, Ohio. A spin-off company, Photonic Developments LLC, makes these products available on a website: www.sleeplamps.com.

When a new mother gets up during the night to care for her baby, she can put on the glasses before turning on an ordinary light bulb. When she is in the nursery or bathroom that is equipped with the new light bulbs, she may safely remove the glasses. Newborn babies do not produce a lot of melatonin, but avoiding suppression of what they have will help them sleep better as well. If the mother is breastfeeding her baby, both she and her baby can benefit from the mother using the glasses a few hours before her normal bedtime. This will maximize her melatonin. Her melatonin will appear in her breast milk and help the baby sleep well.

By avoiding melatonin suppression and the resulting loss of sleep and disruption of her circadian rhythm, she can reduce the risk of postpartum depression. Tests with new mothers to establish the benefits of blocking blue light have been started. There is no need to wait for the result of these tests for new mothers to avoid a possible hazard. Lamps for use in the nursery are now available that will not cause melatonin suppression. It's a way of going back to the benefits of the longer periods of darkness that existed when the human race evolved.

ADHD Improved Without Drugs

Summary Advancing the circadian rhythm has been shown to improve both objective and subjective measures of ADHD symptoms. University scientists have developed special glasses that block the blue rays that cause a delay in the start of the flow of melatonin, the sleep hormone. Putting on the glasses a couple of hours ahead of bedtime eliminates this delay, thereby advancing the circadian rhythm.

University Heights, OH, February 6, 2007 PRWebb: Recent studies at the University of Toronto have shown that moving the start of the flow of melatonin to an earlier hour resulted in a marked improvement in both objective and subjective measures of ADHD symptoms. Twenty-nine adults with DSM-4 ADHD were studied in a 3-week trial. Primary outcome measures included percent reduction on the Brown Adult ADD Scale and the Conner's Adult ADHD Scale. The strongest correlation was between improvement in these scores and the advance in the circadian rhythm.

Scientists at John Carroll University working in the Lighting Innovations Institute have discovered a means to advance the circadian rhythm without the use of any drugs or the bright lights used in the above mentioned study. There is concern that using the lights to advance the circadian rhythm may have the potential to damage the retina. The new approach developed at JCU is to block the blue component in ordinary light that causes delay in the start of the melatonin flow. Normally it doesn't start until after the individual goes into darkness.

By wearing blue-blocking glasses a couple of hours before bedtime, the melatonin can begin to flow at an earlier hour. This is the advance in the circadian rhythm that gave the marked improvement of symptoms of ADHD. An alternative to the blue-blocking glasses has been developed in the form of light bulbs with coatings that block the blue light. Instead of putting on glasses, the individual may simply turn off ordinary lights and turn on the ones with the filters that remove the blue rays. Major use of these devices has been to provide better sleep, avoid postpartum depression, avoid SAD, and reduce the risk of cancer. A spin-off company makes these new products available on the website www.lowbluelights.com.

Contact Richard L. Hansler, Ph.D.
216 397 1657.

In the spring of 2006, we contacted a John Carroll University student, Kim Burkhart, who was then a junior psychology major. She found the glasses were very helpful to her in relieving headaches and helping her sleep. She agreed to prepare for a clinical trial of the glasses as part of her requirements for her psychology degree. Her professor, Dr. John Yost, agreed. She prepared all the paper work with the hope of getting quick approval from the JCU Internal Review Board (IRB).

At the last minute the IRB decided they didn't have authority since they decided the glasses were medical devices. Fortunately, Dr. Briones agreed to act as her sponsor and got the IRB at St.Vincent Charity Hospital to approve her study. Because of the late start, she was not able to get as many patients as she would have liked. It was a double blind study in which the placebo glasses were light yellow and only blocked a small fraction of the light causing melatonin suppression. She found a significant improvement in subjective sleep quality and number of times awakening during the night when using the real glasses for a couple of hours before bedtime.

Dr. Jim Phelps, a M.D. psychiatrist practicing in Corvallis, Oregon, had been working with patients with rapid cycling bipolar disorder. He was aware of earlier studies of a treatment in which patients were placed in darkness for twelve hours at night. The method was successful in calming the cycling, but patients were not willing to endure the treatment.

At some point he heard about our glasses that produce "virtual darkness." The initial results were encouraging, and he gradually accumulated enough experience that he decided to publish the results, which are reproduced in part here with his permission.

Dark therapy for Bipolar Disorder using amber lenses for blue light blockade

James Phelps, M.D.[1]
PsychEducation.org, Corvallis, OR; Corvallis Psychiatric Clinic, Corvallis, OR

Abstract

Many medical illnesses are affected by circadian rhythms. A treatment which could help correct disorganized circadian rhythms would be useful in a broad variety of conditions. One illness in which such a treatment could be easily investigated is Bipolar Disorder, where increasing evidence suggests a central role for circadian rhythms in the etiology of this disorder, at least in some patients. Whereas light therapy has antidepressant effects in some forms of depression, preliminary evidence suggests that darkness may have opposite effects, serving as a mood stabilizer like lithium in some forms of Bipolar Disorder. In a separate line of research, a third human photoreceptor (in addition to rods and cones) has recently been discovered, and fibers from which connect not to the visual cortex but to the biological clock in the hypothalamus.

This photoreceptor is stimulated only by light in the blue portion of the visual spectrum (around 460 nm).

Amber-tinted safety glasses, which block transmission of these wavelengths, have already been shown to preserve normal nocturnal melatonin levels in a light environment which otherwise completely suppresses melatonin production. Therefore it may be possible to influence human circadian rhythms by using these lenses at night to blunt the impact of electric light, particularly the blue light of ubiquitous television screens; in other words, providing a "virtual darkness" instead of the complete darkness studied so far in Bipolar Disorder. One way to investigate this would be to provide the lenses to patients with severe sleep disturbance of probable circadian origin. A preliminary case series herein demonstrates that some patients with Bipolar Disorder experience reduced sleep-onset latency with this approach, suggesting a circadian effect. If amber lenses can effectively simulate darkness, a broad range of conditions might respond to this inexpensive therapeutic tool: common forms of insomnia; sleep deprivation in nursing mothers; circadian rhythm disruption in shift workers; and perhaps even some of the most difficult-to-treat forms of Bipolar Disorder. Randomized trials are warranted.

The author's subjective assessment of patient response (Clinical Global Improvement Scale, CGI) is shown in Table 1.

Table 1. Consecutive patients' response to amber lenses for initial insomnia

CGI	*N*	*%*
3 Very Much Improved	9	42
2 Much Improved	1	5
1 Slightly Improved	1	5
0 No Response	8	38
-1 Slightly Worse	1	5
-2 Much Worse	1	5
-3 Very Much Worse	0	0

Dr. Phelps recommends our glasses on his excellent, informative website www.psycheducation.org. Many of our sales are the result of this recommendation. Some of our strongest testimonials have been from bipolar patients who have been helped by wearing them. Disruption of the circadian rhythm (clock) has been known to be linked to depression.

Marty Alpert joined our group in early 2007. He is an M.D. but has not practiced for a number of years. He has been a successful entrepreneur in the field of computers. He felt that what was holding us back was a lack of clinical trials of the glasses. The study Kim had done was with only a small number of patients. The first study launched was for helping to relive the symptoms of postpartum depression (ppd). Dr. Shoshana Bennett, who had ppd herself, is doing the clinical trial of our glasses and lights. She has written a couple of books on ppd, *Beyond the Blues* and *Postpartum Depression for Dummies.* She is also an active participant in Postpartum Support International. The study is a double blind study where neither the mothers nor Dr. Bennett know which patients have the real thing and which the placebo (lightly tinted) glasses and light bulbs.

A study of the possible benefits for Fibromyalgia patients has been started, with Dr. Harold Bowersox in charge of evaluating the patients. He and his wife, Karen Bowersox, have also written a book, *The Bowersox Protocol for Fibromyalgia and Chronic Fatigue,* on their method of treating FM. Again, it is a double blind study of patients whose primary complaint is insomnia.

Two doctors at University Hospitals (of Cleveland), John Lavin, M.D. and Carl Weitman, M.D. are starting a study of the possible benefit to young people with Attention Deficit and Hyperactivity Disorder (ADHD). They will not be using placebo devices since they have some objective measure of how the patients are doing and will compare these measures before and after using the devices.

When all these tests are complete, we will be in a position to know just how effective blocking blue light in the evening can be. We will then be in a position to work with the medical community without being challenged.

The really big question, of course, is whether the risk of cancer can be reduced by maximizing melatonin and the other hormones the pineal gland produces that may be even better cancer fighters. There is at least one paper that suggests they are better than melatonin by itself. Tests to determine the effectiveness of maximizing pineal hormones will require many years. One way to speed up the trials is to use patients that are cancer survivors and are therefore at higher risk than the general population. Patients who decline to be part of the test could serve as controls. The glasses would be utilized in concert with whatever other treatment is used. Some bookkeeping and the cost of the glasses and educating the patients would be the only costs. This is such a simple thing to do. We may be able to convince someone to do it, if the trails now going on continue to come out positive.

In the meantime, those who are at high risk for cancer and others who simply want to sleep better don't have to wait for clinical trials.

CHAPTER 17.

Examining the Evidence That Controlling Light Can Cut the Risk of Cancer

Most of us are skeptics. Maybe what we said about light at night and cancer in Chapter 1 is true, but how much evidence do we really have that using light at night increases the risk of cancer? Our objective here is to carefully look at that evidence. Among the most convincing pieces of evidence are the studies of the effect of long days and short nights done with animals. The hours of light and dark (LD) are abbreviated, e.g. "16:8" is sixteen hours of light and eight hours of darkness. Because the reader may want to go to www.pubmed.gov to look up these abstracts, we have given the year and the author's last name and first initials to help locate the article.

The first article turned up on a PubMed search for "continuous light animals" is a 1969 series of six papers by Singh in which polycystic ovarian disease is shown to be the result of exposure to continuous light. Continuous light results in persistent estrus (ready to breed) due to disruption of the normal cycle in the production of hormones. Polycystic ovarian disease can lead to cancer.

A 1975 paper by Kuralasov, A.K. found that, in darkness, the transplanting of rat mammary carcinoma was successful a smaller percentage of the time and the growth was delayed. The presence of melatonin when the surgery was done in darkness may have been responsible.

A 1978 paper by Cohen, M. et al. points out five conditions that suggest that reduced pineal secretion (mostly melatonin) increases the risk of cancer. 1) Pineal calcification is most common in countries with high rates of breast cancer, 2) Chlorpromazine raises serum melatonin; there are reports that psychiatric patients taking it have a lower incidence of breast cancer, 3) the pineal and melatonin may influence tumor induction and growth in experimental animals, 4) the demonstration of a melatonin receptor in the human ovary suggests a direct influence of this hormone on the ovarian function and possibly oestrogen production, 5) impaired pineal secretion is believed to be an important factor triggering abnormally early puberty (early menarche is a risk factor for breast cancer).

A 1982 paper in "Cancer Letters" by Kothare L.S., Shah P.N., and Mhatre M.C., entitled "Effect of continuous light on the incidence of 9, 10dimethyl-1, 2-benzanthracene induced mammary tumors in female Holtzman rats," reported that the incidence of adenocarcinoma in rats raised under continuous light was 95% compared to 60% for rats raised under a more normal LD of 10:14.The difference was attributed to the lack of function by the pineal gland caused by continuous light. In subsequent experiments, this group found that surgically removing the pineal gland resulted in the same effect on tumor development as continuous light. They further found that supplementing with melatonin reduced the cancer rate, but not as effectively as having a pineal gland and having more normal lighting conditions of LD 10:14 that did not suppress melatonin completely. Supplementing these rats with melatonin further reduced the cancer rate.

A 1983 paper by Stanberry, L.R. et al. found that eighteen-hour nights increased the time for tumors to start and decreased tumor growth rate in hamsters. They concluded (in part) that the quantity, time, and duration of melatonin presentation all had an important effect on tumor growth.

A 1989 paper by Barni, S. et al. found that the melatonin concentration was highest in breast cancer patients with the best prognosis. Mean levels of melatonin were significantly higher in estrogen receptor positive patients than in negative ones. They concluded that melatonin plays a role in the hormone dependency of human breast cancer.

In the "Journal of Biological Rhythms" 1994 winter edition, Nelson R.J. and Blom J.M., published (in part) the following abstract:

"Adult female deer mice (*Peromyscus maniculatus*) were housed in either long (LD 16:8) or short (LD 8:16) days for 8 weeks, then injected with the chemical carcinogen 9,10-dimethyl-1,2-benzanthracene (DMBA) dissolved in dimethyl sulfoxide (DMSO) or with the DMSO vehicle alone. Animals were evaluated weekly for 8 weeks after injection. None of the animals treated with DMSO developed tumors in any of the experiments. Nearly 90% of the long-day deer mice injected with DMBA developed squamous cell carcinoma. None of the short-day deer mice injected with DMBA developed tumors. Small lesions developed at the site of injection; short-day females had less severe lesions and healed faster than long-day females."

To sum this up, in case you couldn't decipher all the lingo, the mice were given a chemical injection of a material that causes cancer. Almost all of the mice developed cancer when kept under sixteen hours of light and eight hours of darkness each day. *None of the mice developed cancer when kept under only eight hours of light and sixteen hours of darkness.* Long periods of darkness, when melatonin may be present, resulted in preventing the development of cancer, even though a carcinogen was administered.

In a related study of the same type of mice, Nelson, R.J. and Demas, G.E. found "These results confirm that both male and female deer mice housed in short days [had] enhanced immune function relative to long-day animals."

In 1997, Li, J.C. reported the results of a study of constantly shifting (every three days) the hours of light and dark (LD) from 14:10 to 10:14. Among other negative effects on health, he found that carcinoma tumors grew faster on the shifted animals than on ones kept in a constant 14:10 condition. It was concluded that constantly shifting the schedule resulted in less melatonin being produced.

A 2000 study by Anderson et al. found continuous light significantly increased the incidence of carcinogen-induced tumors in rats compared to rats raised under LD of 8:16.

A 2001 study by Beniashvili, D.S. et al. found that the cancer rate among offspring of female rats given a carcinogen during their pregnancy was much higher among rats raised in constant light, medium for rats raised in LD of 12:12, and much lower in rates raised in continual darkness. Evidently the carcinogen passes on to the offspring but can be canceled out by the young spending longer time in darkness (when melatonin can be present).

In a 2003 study by Blask, D.F. et al., the rate of growth of human breast cancer grafts increased markedly under continuous light compared to under a light dark routine.

A 2004 study of chicken hens by Moore, C.B. and Siopes, T.D. found that ovarian tumors grew rapidly in LD 16:8 but shrank in LD 8:16. This is quite amazing. All that was changed were the hours of darkness and the tumors went away.

A 2004 study by Ferreira, A.C. et al. found the melatonin output from the pineal gland in rats with carcinosarcoma increased by three times compared to controls within fourteen days after tumor implantation. This rise in melatonin production as a result of the presence of cancer might explain why some studies have wrongly concluded there was no correlation between low melatonin output and incidence of cancer.

To summarize, all these studies (mostly with animals) show that tumors grow in long periods of light and don't grow, or grow slowly, or actually shrink in long periods of darkness. The main difference appears to be the amount or duration of melatonin. To my knowledge, no reversals in which tumor growth was more rapid when melatonin was present were reported.

These are truly amazing results. All that is changed is the duration of light or, more significantly, the duration of darkness, the hours when melatonin may be present. One would think, knowing all this, that cancer research groups would be trying similar experiments with humans. To my knowledge, only one group (Lissoni, P. et al.) in Italy as early as 1989 began trying melatonin along with other treatments for cancer, based on the results of the animal studies. I have not been able to locate any studies where extending the time in darkness was tried with human cancer patients. Considering the ease and lack of any cost, one would think that someone would have tried this.

To this day, the only use of darkness therapy of which I am aware is the work of Jim Phelps, M.D., psychiatrist, who is using it to treat rapid cycling bipolar disorder, described in an earlier chapter. He has an excellent website, www.psycheducation.org. With the huge amount of time and money being spent on cancer research, one would think someone would try keeping patients in darkness for sixteen hours a day. It would cost nothing. Better yet, use blue-blocking glasses to create "virtual darkness" for part of the time.

But one can argue that these are mostly animal studies, many of which were conducted on nocturnal animals, in which the presence of melatonin resulted in the animal becoming active rather than going to sleep. Even in nocturnal animals melatonin is still suppressed by light.

In fact, very low levels of light (0.2 lux) can cause changes in rats. Just the light leaking under a door may be enough to cause increased tumor growth, according to a 1997 paper by Dauchy, R.T. et al.

Rather than extending the use of prolonged darkness to treat cancer patients, the result of extended periods of darkness became known in a different way. Blind people are in continual darkness.The 1991 paper by Hahn, R.A. concerned the incidence of breast cancer in blind women compared to their sighted counterparts. He found the incidence for the blind women was about half that of sighted women. In a French paper in 1992, Coleman and others suggested that a study of breast cancer incidence in blind women should be done.

Also in a 1992 paper, Stevens and others suggested that the high rate of breast cancer in industrialized countries compared to primitive societies is due to the use of electricity to produce light at night or electromagnet fields (EMF) themselves.

A 1993 paper by Reiter states there is evidence that changing magnetic fields as well as light can reduce melatonin production that might increase the risk of cancer.

In 1996, Stevens presented what he calls the "Melatonin Hypothesis," that light at night suppresses melatonin production and that EMF may also suppress melatonin and this is the reason for the higher incidence of breast cancer.

A 1998 study by Feychting, M et al. done in Sweden showed totally blind people had approximately two-thirds the risk of cancer of all types in both men and women than sighted people.

A 1999 study by Kukala et al. done in Finland showed the incidence of all cancers for totally blind men was more than twice as great as for society in general.The higher smoking rate among blind men was considered to be a possible explanation. On the other hand, a second paper described a lower rate of breast cancer among blind women in Finland.

In a 1999 German study reported by Erren, "Consistent with our prediction, epidemiological data indicate uniformly low risks for hormone-dependent cancers in the Arctic." This is based on the melatonin hypothesis that long periods of darkness are beneficial. In countries such as Sweden, where electric lights illuminate the long, dark nights, the cancer rate is not low. The cancer rate is low among the Inuit of northern Canada, who do not have electric lighting.

Also in 1999, Dr. George Brainard of Thomas Jefferson University in Philadelphia did a review of all the evidence that light at night and subsequent melatonin suppression might be the source of the elevated rate of cancer in advanced societies. He concluded there is sufficient evidence that more studies were warranted. He has gone on to become the foremost researcher in this field.

In 2000, Bartsch, H. published the results of the effect of melatonin and another pineal extract on cell cultures from seven ovarian cancers and seven breast cancers. Melatonin inhibited the growth of some, but not all, of the cultures. The pineal extract inhibited the growth of all of them. When we speak of natural or endogenous melatonin, we probably need to remind everyone that we are including other unidentified hormones produced by the pineal gland. These other hormones appear to be more powerful cancer fighters than melatonin by itself. This may explain why giving melatonin by mouth has not become a widely accepted therapy for cancer.

A 2001 study in Norway by Kliukliene et al. showed blind women had a significantly lower breast cancer rate. This study considered more than 15,000 women.

In 2001, two milestone papers showed that the blue component in white light is responsible for suppression of melatonin. This was discussed in detail in an earlier chapter.

A study done in 2001 at Harvard by Czeisler found that blind and sighted individuals produced melatonin for nine to eleven hours if the sighted individuals were kept in darkness. This suggests that being in darkness longer than eleven hours will not result in any further significant increase in melatonin. He did not consider other output of the pineal gland.

In 2001, a Japanese paper described the result of a study of melatonin suppression in patients with delayed sleep phase syndrome, or DSPS. For a given exposure to light, the DSPS patients showed a significantly greater suppression of melatonin than the controls. This suggests that those with DSPS are likely to have a greater risk of cancer associated with use of light at night.

In a 2002 paper by Glickman (a colleague of Brainard) he states, "Under highly controlled exposure circumstances, less than 1 lux of monochromatic light elicited a significant suppression of nocturnal melatonin."

In 2002, Poole summed up an international symposium on light, endocrine systems, and cancer with the belief that both epidemiologic and laboratory studies in this area are expected to grow appreciably in scope and scale.

A 2002 paper by Stevens documents the five-fold difference between cancer rates in primitive societies and industrialized societies. He raises the question of whether light at night is the likely cause.

In another 2002 paper, Anisimov in Russia writes, "The role of the modulation of the pineal gland function in development of cancer is discussed in the review. An inhibition of the pineal function with pinealectomy or with the exposure to the constant light regimen stimulates mammary carcinogenesis, whereas the light deprivation inhibits the carcinogenesis. Epidemiological observations on increased risk of breast cancer in nightshift workers, flight attendants, radio and telegraph operators, and on decreased risk in blind women are in accordance with the results of experiments in rodents. Treatment with pineal indole hormone melatonin inhibits carcinogenesis in pinealectomized rats or animals kept at the standard light/dark regimen (LD) or at the constant illumination (LL) regimen."

In another 2002 paper, Reiter examined the damaging effect of exposure to light at inappropriate times, namely when we should be producing melatonin. He argued that reducing the antioxidant effects of melatonin leads to more DNA damage that leads to cancer development.

In an important paper in 2003, Blask and Brainard and others described the growth of human cancer cells transplanted into rats. Under constant light conditions that minimized melatonin, the tumors grew rapidly, while under normal light-dark conditions that allowed melatonin to flow during the dark periods, the tumors grew only very slowly. This was the first direct biological evidence for a potential link between constant light exposure and increased human breast cancer.

In 2003, Anisimov added to his earlier comments that "Pineal peptide preparation Epithalamin and synthetic tetrapeptide Epitalon (Ala-Glu-Asp-Gly) are potent inhibitors of mammary carcinogenesis in rodents and might be useful in the prevention of breast cancer in women at risk."

In 2003, Schernhammer and others from Harvard extended their study of the effect of nightshift work to colorectal cancer. They found that working rotating shifts for many years increased the risk of that cancer as well as breast cancer.

A French study in 2003 by Filipski et al. found, "Tumor growth was faster in mice with lesioned suprachiasmatic nucleus (SCN) (site of internal clock) than in controls (undamaged SCN) for both tumor models studied, Glasgow osteosarcoma (GOS) and pancreatic adenocarcinoma."

In a 2004 paper, Pauley states that "lighting has become a public health issue." This is based on his examination of the evidence to that date.

In a 2004 paper, Schernhammer et al. ask the question, "Melatonin and cancer risk: does light at night compromise physiologic cancer protection by lowering serum melatonin levels?" She provides the answer, "We hypothesize that the potential primary culprit for this observed association is the lack of melatonin, a cancer-protective agent whose production is severely diminished in people exposed to light at night."

The French team under the leadership of Filipski published a 2004 paper, "The Effects of Chronic Jet Lag on Tumor Progression in Mice." They found "Tumors grew faster in the jet-lagged animals as compared with controls (ANOVA, P < 0.001), whereas exposure to constant light or darkness had no effect (ANOVA, P = 0.66 and P = 0.8, respectively)." ANOVA is a software analysis program that provides a measure of the cause and effect relationship. Low P is a strong relationship. The chronic jet lag was provided by advancing the 12:12 light-dark cycle by eight hours every two days.

In 2005, a Finish study by Verkasalo, P.K. et al. showed women who consistently slept unusually long (nine hours or more) had about one-fourth the rate of breast cancer as women who consistently slept seven hours or less. A study of data on nurses in the United States done by Schernhammer, E. et al. in 2006 found no similar evidence for any benefit to sleeping a long time.

A 2005 Canadian paper by Knight, J. A. et al. found positive correlation between duration of exercise and amount of melatonin produced in overnight urine. This is suggested as a mechanism by which exercise reduces the risk of breast cancer.

The Finish group reported in 2006 that the study of hormone-related cancers (breast and prostate) in blind and visually impaired persons showed a lower incidence while other cancers did not.

Schernhammer, E. et al. reported in 2005 that the incidence of breast cancer was significantly lower in women who had a higher concentration of melatonin in their first morning urine.

Perhaps the most convincing evidence of the importance of melatonin in reducing breast cancer risk comes from the study by Brainard, Blask et al. reported in 2005. In this study, they took samples of blood from women volunteers under three conditions: during the day when no melatonin was present, at night in darkness when melatonin was present, and at night, but after exposure to light so no melatonin was present. Human breast cancer tumors grown on the backs of rats were supplied with these three different types of blood. With the type that contained melatonin, the tumors either showed no growth or very slow growth. With the two types without melatonin the tumors grew rapidly. The compelling results of these experiments led the head of the National Institute of Environmental Health Sciences to issue this press release.

FOR IMMEDIATE RELEASE

December 19, 2005

Results from a new study in laboratory mice show that nighttime exposure to artificial light stimulated the growth of human breast tumors by suppressing the levels of a key hormone called melatonin. The study also showed that extended periods of nighttime darkness greatly slowed the growth of these tumors.

The study results might explain why female nightshift workers have a higher rate of breast cancer. It also offers a promising new explanation for the epidemic rise in breast cancer incidence in industrialized countries like the United States.

The National Cancer Institute and the National Institute of Environmental Health Sciences, agencies of the federal National Institutes of Health, provided funding to researchers at the Bassett Research Institute of the Mary Imogene Bassett Hospital in Cooperstown, New York and the Thomas Jefferson University in Philadelphia, Pa. The results are published in the December 1, 2005 issue of the scientific journal Cancer Research.

"This is the first experimental evidence that artificial light plays an integral role in the growth of human breast cancer," said NIEHS Director David A. Schwartz, M.D. "This finding will enable scientists to develop new strategies for evaluating the effects of light and other environmental factors on cancer growth."

"The risk of developing breast cancer is about five times higher in industrialized nations than it is in underdeveloped countries," said Les Reinlib, Ph.D., a program administrator with the NIEHS' grants division. "These results suggest that the increasing nighttime use of electric lighting, both at home and in the workplace, may be a significant factor."

Previous research showed that artificial light suppresses the brain's production of melatonin, a hormone that helps to regulate a person's sleeping and waking cycles. The new study shows that melatonin also plays a key role in the development of cancerous tumors.

"We know that many tumors are largely dependent on a nutrient called linoleic acid, an essential fatty acid, in order to grow," said David Blask, M.D., Ph.D., a neuroendocrinologist with the Bassett Research Institute and lead author on the study. "Melatonin interferes with the tumor's ability to use linoleic acid as a growth signal, which causes tumor metabolism and growth activity to shut down."

To test this hypothesis, the researchers injected human breast cancer cells into laboratory mice. Once these cells developed into cancerous tumors, the tumors were implanted into female rats where they could continue to grow and develop.

The researchers then took blood samples from 12 healthy, premenopausal volunteers. The samples were collected under three different conditions – during the daytime, during the nighttime following 2 hours of complete darkness, and during the nighttime following 90 minutes of exposure to bright fluorescent light. These blood samples were then pumped directly through the developing tumors.

"The melatonin-rich blood collected from subjects while in total darkness severely slowed the growth of the tumors. These results are due to a direct effect of the melatonin on the cancer cells," said Blask. "The melatonin is clearly suppressing tumor development and growth."

In contrast, tests with the melatonin-depleted blood from light-exposed subjects stimulated tumor growth. "We observed rapid growth comparable to that seen with administration of daytime blood samples, when tumor activity is particularly high," Blask said.

According to the researchers, melatonin exerts a strong influence on the body's circadian rhythm, an internal biological clock that regulates sleep-wake cycle, body temperature, endocrine functions, and a number of disease processes including heart attack, stroke and asthma. "Evidence is emerging that disruption of one's circadian clock is associated with cancer in humans, and that interference with internal timekeeping can tip the balance in favor of tumor development," said Blask.

"The effects we are seeing are of greatest concern to people who routinely stay in a lighted environment during times when they would prefer to be sleeping," said Mark Rollag, Ph.D., a visiting research scientist at the University of Virginia and one of the study co-authors. "This is because melatonin concentrations are not elevated during a person's normal waking hours."

"If the link between light exposure and cancer risk can be confirmed, it could have an immediate impact on the production and use of artificial lighting in this country," said Blask. "This might include lighting with a wavelength and intensity that does not disrupt melatonin levels and internal timekeeping.

"Day workers who spend their time indoors would benefit from lighting that better mimics sunlight," added Blask. "Companies that employ shift workers could introduce lighting that allows the workers to see without disrupting their circadian and melatonin rhythms."

NIEHS, a component of the National Institutes of Health, supports research to understand the effects of the environment on human health. For more information on breast cancer and other environmental health topics, visit http://www.niehs.nih.gov/home.htm

End of Press Release

A 2006 study by Kubo, T. et al. from Japan found that men who worked rotating shifts had a very significantly increased risk of prostate cancer than those who worked on non-rotating shifts. This was based on a study that included over 14,000 subjects of whom thirty-one developed prostate cancer.

A 2006 study by Lie, J. A. et al. of Norwegian nurses found a large increase (2.2 times) in the risk of developing breast cancer in women who had worked nights for thirty or more years compared to nurses who had not worked nights.

A 2006 study by Buja, A. et al. of female flight attendants found a statistically significant elevation of risk for melanoma and breast cancer.

A 2006 study by Feychting, M. et al. found no evidence of a link between electromagnetic field exposure and breast cancer.

In a 2007 paper by Kayumov, L. et al. entitled "Prevention of melatonin suppression by nocturnal lighting: relevance to cancer," melatonin levels in subjects were measured under 800 lux white light with and without a filter that blocked blue light below 530nm. The filtered light allowed 92% melatonin production compared to that observed in very dim light. This was published in the "European Journal of Cancer Prevention."

What, then, can we conclude from all this? There is no direct proof that using light at night causes cancer. It does appear that suppressing melatonin (and possibly other pineal secretions) by using light at night can allow tumors to grow. At least one study showed that taking melatonin was not as effective as preserving one's own pineal secretions.

What action do these results suggest? Getting back to the schedule of light and dark under which we evolved seems to me a logical conclusion. While actual darkness may still be better than virtual darkness obtained by blocking blue light, wearing blue-blocking glasses for a few hours before bedtime, to give a combined period of darkness of eleven hours, seems like a practical way to minimize the risk of cancer, or at least of breast, ovarian, and prostate cancer.

CHAPTER 18.

The Next Generation Of Light Bulbs

A strong impetus for starting this whole venture was the concern that ordinary light bulbs, used in the hours before bedtime, were literally killing people. They were preventing the flow of the cancer-fighting hormone melatonin. Having spent more than fifty years developing better and brighter light bulbs (with lots of blue light), I felt a sense of responsibility to do something about it. We set out to develop light bulbs that did not produce blue light, and did so with some success. The problem is that these light bulbs produce yellow-orange light. What we would like to do is make lights that appear white but which don't produce blue light.

The color of light is a tricky subject. The eye is amazing in so many ways, and how it perceives color is one of the most amazing. Dr. Land, the inventor of the Polaroid camera, was able to demonstrate full color slides using only two colors of light. While I never really understood how that was possible, I do know that many optical illusions exploit the eye-brain ability to create a belief that something is real that is only illusion.

One principle of color is that of complementary colors. One can take light of one color and mix it with light of its complement, and if the ratio of intensities is right, the resulting mixture will appear white. If that light is used to illuminate a color palette, many of the colors will appear very strange. We say its color rendering is poor. However, our experience is that the eye (brain) is quite good at believing familiar objects of a known color appear surprisingly normal.

In any event, the possibility of making light bulbs without blue light that appear white can make use of this principle. Fortunately at this point in human history, there is great interest in improving the efficiency of lighting and also of getting rid of mercury in our light bulbs. Light emitting diodes are being developed very rapidly that have improved efficiency and higher output. They are also available in a range of colors.

The reason our non-blue light producing light bulbs appear yellow is that yellow is the complement of blue. To get back to light that appears white we need to also remove the yellow light. If we do this, we are left with red and green light which, when mixed in the right ratio, appears white. Rather than starting with white light and removing blue and yellow, we can start with red and green LEDs and mix their light. This is the approach we are using in trying to create lights that have high efficiency and appear white but are free of the damaging blue light that suppresses melatonin.

Part of the problem of using such lights is that they may result in melatonin being produced too early in the evening. For this reason we are working on an approach where normal white LEDs are used in the early evening. A built-in clock will switch to the red and green LEDs at a selected time. These lamps will initially be expensive, but the cost will gradually come down. Light bulbs that appear white but which do not suppress melatonin in the hours before bedtime and that produce a full spectrum the rest of the time will soon be a reality.

There is no logical end to this book. Things are just getting really exciting. So stay in touch for the second edition. In the meantime, maximize your melatonin and enjoy a good night's sleep and relax knowing you are doing something to reduce your risk of cancer.

CHAPTER 19.

Testimonials

For a number of people with serious sleeping problems extending over many years, the response to using the glasses has been enthusiastic.

From an M.D. sleep specialist:

I just sent an e-mail to Dr. Carome letting him know that I have given away the 3 glasses that he gave me, and all 3 patients are now sleeping like babies!! I am in awe!

Your eyewear has made a tremendous difference in my life in only 4 weeks! I am now getting to bed by midnight each night for the first time in 11 years. I felt the effects from wearing your glasses immediately. I started having vivid dreams and slept very soundly. I woke up early each morning and was ready for bed earlier each night.

From a M.D. sleep specialist:

I wanted to share with you that my most challenging insomnia patient was able to sleep a full 5–6 hours consecutively every night he used the glasses. He wants to buy all lights and filters for his house!

My experiment with the glasses turned out remarkably well. I would put the glasses on one hour before bedtime each night. Not only did I fall asleep within 10 minutes of actually trying to fall asleep, I also did not wake up in the middle of the night or only woke up once. This is quite an improvement from my normal sleep pattern.

I use these for reading prior to bedtime and find I get sleepy and am able to initiate sleep at a more appropriate time. If I awake in the middle of the night and have trouble falling asleep again, I wear the glasses and read, rather than worry about sleep, and find I return to sleep more easily than if I read w/o the glasses.

I do find the glasses to be beneficial. They have helped me develop a more structured sleep pattern. My doctor had given me a trial pair, so after my purchase I was able to return his loan of the glasses. He was ready to give them to another patient. I would recommend them to anyone struggling with sleep problems, as an alternative to medicine.

I have been using the glasses during the week but not in the weekends. I can tell you that I noticed a difference when I use them. I get to sleep more or less at the same time every day. When I have been wearing the glasses I have been able to fall asleep easier and to have a better quality of sleep during the night.

I purchased the glasses a month ago and have used them for 2 hours prior to bed every night. I really do think they are helping my sleep!!! I have had a lifetime of sleep problems as well as I am a breast cancer survivor so anything I can try to get more and quality rest I will do. I am very pleased with your glasses and thank you for making them available. What a great option other than a pill!

I did not have any clear need for the glasses (no sleep problems or body clock issues) when I purchased the glasses. I purchased them as a proactive step to minimize blue light effects on my body clock. I have been using the glasses primarily when I use my computer or watch TV at night. I am very pleased with the purchase. I have been measuring my body temperature on days when I wear and don't wear the glasses and so far it appears the amplitude of body temperature rhythm might be greater with use of the glasses—which based upon my knowledge of circadian body temperature I would interpret as an improvement.

I have found the sleep glasses to be of benefit. I use them when I watch TV at night, and I find that I can go right to sleep when I turn the TV off, rather than my previous pattern of being up and somewhat "wired" after watching TV at night. (Not that being able to watch more TV is a good thing necessarily! but it does give me a chance to unwind after a long day.) By the way, I got to your site from psych-education.org, which I found to be a very informative site. I am not bi-polar but I have started using light therapy in the winters for seasonal affective disorder, and his site provided very helpful background references. Best wishes for the continued growth of your product line.

The glasses are a God-send. You can pry my glasses from my cold dead fingers! Occasionally I will forget to get my glasses on and I want to tell you, I am panicked! My wife continues to snore. Before the glasses I might spend one to two nights a week on the couch after being awakened in the middle of the night. The couch misses me! I continue to refer anyone who will listen to your web site. Hope your project is progressing.

I like using the combination of glasses, yellow light bulb in bedside lamp, and yellow night light. I turn them all on around 7PM every evening, and they help me wind down so that by 9PM I can go to bed and get to sleep immediately. They are lifesavers!

I am continuing to wear the glasses. And YES! they do seem to work! I feel tired much earlier in the evening, am sleeping better, and waking earlier! I think the concept brilliant and am very pleased with the investment. We are also using the computer screen (nearly all of the time)... And think this is a wise safety precaution. We are considering also light bulbs throughout the house that have no blue light. Thank you for your work—we have benefited from it greatly!

I love my sleep glasses. I've been wearing them since I received them and I think they are very beneficial to my consistent sleep patterns.

I purchased the light bulbs and they have been wonderful. Please let me know if you need more info.

The glasses do seem to be helping—I use them in the evening to watch TV and then keep them on until in the master bedroom. I also put the amber light bulbs in the master bedroom and the nightlight in the master bath. My sleep seems more natural and deeper, with dreams but not nightmarish dreams (as with swallowing a melatonin tablet). Was previously taking a melatonin lozenge (sublingually to avoid nightmares, which are common with women who use melatonin orally) at bedtime, but now rarely have to use the supplement. Sleeping pills of ANY type just do not work for me and leave me terribly groggy the next day.

I bought your sleep glasses about 5 months ago. I continue to use them nightly. I find I achieve a deeper level of sleep by using them. I can tell this by the way I feel in the morning when I wake up, and by the more vivid and memorable dreams I have when I use them. Interesting to note, I have insulin resistance and I have also noticed on the few occasions when I have not used the glasses, I wake up with more fluid retention, my face is much more puffy, so the glasses clearly have some effect on my blood sugar or insulin or both. Finally, I want to let you know that I was so impressed with your product that I ordered a pair of your sleep glasses for my stepdaughter. She is a college student and tends to keep late hours and she finds she feels much more rested after using the glasses. And I bought my brother the nightlights because he is diabetic and gets up frequently during the night and he feels much more rested now that he avoids using his lights and relies only on the nightlight when he gets up.

I am very happy with the low blue lights sleep glasses. They really help with sleep onset although my insomnia is more of a sleep maintenance problem. I feel more free to look at the computer at night or watch TV without those activities interfering with sleep. I also like the amber light bulb. I use it in my reading lamp at night, so I can read close to bedtime without worrying about melatonin interruption.

The glasses are very helpful and I am wearing them right now as it is nearly 8 pm. A few hours of wearing the sleep glasses really helps me to fall asleep at a reasonable time and to have a better quality of sleep. I am a psychiatrist and I recently purchased an extra pair of sleep glasses to lend out to my patients to try. So far only one has tried it but it helped him to regulate his sleep schedule. I am looking forward to having other patients try it for a week or so each. Then they will order their own glasses.

Yes, I love them. They are definitely working. I am happy to report that my sleep has been increasing over the course of several weeks. Since I have been a chronic non-sleeper for several months on end, I am glad to report that the glasses are effective. Thank you!

Just wanted to write a note of thanks and say GOD BLESS YOU. Your altruistic products have helped my bipolar husband more than any drugs. May and the summer months are always tough as he gets manic. He wore your glasses last night and I noticed he seemed more relaxed, although he wouldn't admit it. Then, when he went to bed I noticed his breathing was much quieter. When he awoke this morning he had actually slept. This is a miracle. Incidentally, my children, who have never been able to get to sleep at a decent hour, are also doing fantastically well and sleeping like clockwork since I installed the lights in their room. This could help anxious kids too, since when I called my doctor he gave me a prescription for some drug to help my 2-year-old sleep (I wouldn't give it to him). I think when you get this more mainstream you will do very well. And the glasses and bulbs are environmentally sound as well.

They really work. If you have trouble falling asleep and staying asleep they help you do both. If you don't have trouble falling or staying asleep they make you have a deeper better sleep.

Dear Founders,

My husband and I want to thank you for the miracle that you have brought to our family. We have four great kids, and our youngest had a terrible time falling asleep at night. Dr. Gonzalez suggested the glasses, and our 6-year-old has been wearing them now for over two months. We noticed a big difference in just 3 days! Prior to using the glasses, our youngest could not fall asleep before 11:30 pm, and he slept until at least 10:30 in the morning. Waking him for school was literally like waking the dead. It was impossible. Now, he falls asleep by 8:30 pm with ease and is eager to wake up for school at 7:00. He is energetic all day.

What a gift you have given to us. My kids are in 4 different schools, and I have started to recommend the glasses to various administrators and teachers because it is a shame for other kids to suffer.

Thank you! Keep up the research!

End of testimonials

Admittedly not all users of blue-blocking glasses and light bulbs have found them helpful. Those people who make very little melatonin are obviously not going to be helped by not suppressing it. If there is nothing to suppress, not suppressing it has no meaning. Other people whose circadian clocks don't function normally may require more than glasses or light bulbs to help them.

I hope the reader enjoyed the book. Without action, knowledge has little value.

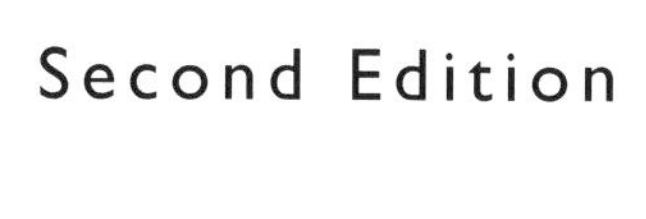

Second Edition

CHAPTER 1A

Cutting the Risk of Cancer

Perhaps my biggest disappointment following the publication of *Great Sleep! Reduced Cancer!* has been the lack of interest in the prevention of cancer by the "Cancer Industry." The nonprofit foundations that raise money for cancer research are only interested in supporting research that is looking for a cure. That apparently is where the money is, not in prevention. The only group I'm aware of that is actually doing prevention work is the Cancer Prevention Institute of California. Much of this group's work is in educating people about potential harm from unwanted chemicals in the environment. It does not have the resources to carry out a clinical trial of avoiding light at night as a way of reducing cancer.

The National Institutes of Health is funding some cancer prevention studies that are primarily focused on food, e.g., lycopene found in tomatoes. It has funded some studies that have shown that melatonin reduces the rate of cancer growth, so it is likely NIH will eventually look at what controls the amount of melatonin produced (light at night).

My book *Heroes of Cancer Prevention Research* (2012) has not reached the *New York Times* best seller list but is gradually increasing in sales. Hopefully this mention of it will spark your interest. I'm running an ad for it in *Coping*, the cancer magazine you see in doctors' waiting rooms.

The most exciting recent news regarding breast cancer concerns metastasis. Metastasis of cancer to distant sites is the thing that kills most cancer patients, not the original tumor. A breakthrough study (2012) at Tulane and at Thomas Jefferson Medical Schools showed that the increased risk of metastasis of both breast cancer and prostate cancer can result from disrupting the circadian (daily) cycle, causing loss of melatonin due to exposure to light at night.

The study examined the molecular processes involved in the transition of stable cancer cells into cancer cells capable of moving through the bloodstream to distant sites where new tumors can develop. The researchers examined how the presence of various compounds required for the different steps in the process were associated with the presence or absence of melatonin. They looked at this in both cultured cancer cells (both breast cancer and prostate cancer) and also in human cancers grown as grafts on the backs of rats but supplied with human blood. In every case, cancer cells retained a static structure when melatonin was present; however, in the absence of melatonin, the conditions necessary for metastasis to occur were observed.

This study provides an incentive for women who have breast cancer (and men who have prostate cancer) to do everything they can to maximize the natural output of the pineal gland, which includes not only melatonin but other cancer-fighting hormones.

The first studies using cancer tumors grown as grafts on rats and fed with human blood had been completed just prior to the publication of the first edition. Since then, a number of studies of additional types of cancers have been made using this method. The results have confirmed the earlier studies and demonstrated the benefit of maximizing melatonin.

Partly as a result of these studies, a number of the scientists conducting the studies have authored the strongest paper yet blaming ordinary lighting for the rise in the incidence of breast cancer. I am including the entire abstract of the study, which was published on December 24, 2013 in *CA: A Cancer Journal for Clinicians* under the title "Breast Cancer and Circadian Disruption from Electric Lighting in the Modern World."

Abstract

Breast cancer is the leading cause of cancer death among women worldwide, and there is only a limited explanation of why. Risk is highest in the most industrialized countries but also is rising rapidly in the developing world. Known risk factors account for only a portion of the incidence in the high-risk populations, and there has been considerable speculation and many false leads on other possibly major determinants of risk, such as dietary fat. A hallmark of industrialization is the increasing use of electricity to light the night, both within the home and without. It has only recently become clear that this evolutionarily new and, thereby, unnatural exposure can disrupt human circadian rhythmicity, of which three salient features are melatonin production, sleep, and the circadian clock. A convergence of research in cells, rodents, and humans suggests that the health consequences of circadian disruption may be substantial. An innovative experimental model has shown that light at night markedly increases the growth of human breast cancer xenografts in rats. In humans, the theory that light exposure at night increases breast cancer risk leads to specific predictions that are being tested epidemiologically: evidence has accumulated on risk in shift workers, risk in blind women, and the impact of sleep duration on risk. If electric light at night does explain a portion of the breast cancer burden, then there are practical interventions that can be implemented, including more selective use of light and the adoption of recent advances in lighting technology and application. CA Cancer J Clin 2013. © 2013 American Cancer Society, Inc.

This paper is very encouraging for me in that it vindicates our work of providing a means to avoid the circadian disruption caused by the use of white light at night. It justifies the use of amber glasses (or light bulbs free of the blue wavelengths) by anyone wishing to reduce the risk of cancer. The paper is also encouraging because it is published through the American Cancer Society. At last this organization is taking notice. Some time ago, I talked with someone at the American Cancer Society who did indicate an awareness of the melatonin-suppressing ability of light at night, but she declined to give an address where I could mail a copy of the first edition of this book.

In addition to the research study on breast cancer and exposure to electric light at night discussed above, there have been several other recent studies with findings related to the connection between melatonin and cancer.

A January 2014 paper from Sao Paulo and Detroit using human triple negative breast cancer xenografts found that melatonin prevented the development of blood vessels, thus preventing the tumors from growing and metastasizing. This is part of the evidence that melatonin is beneficial in all types of cancer, not only those stimulated by estrogen.

Some very recent studies by Mariana Figueiro of the Lighting Research Center at Rensselaer Polytechnic Institute indicate that children's eyes are more sensitive to light than adults' when it comes to melatonin suppression. This is disturbing because early maturation of children is correlated with reduced melatonin production. (Tumors in the hypothalamus that prevent the production of melatonin by the pineal gland result in precocious puberty in very young boys and girls, e.g., five years old). Early maturation in girls is correlated with an increased risk for breast cancer in later life.

A recent paper from India describes a possible mechanism by which melatonin has this effect on maturation:

> *"The pineal gland influences human reproductive function at hypothalamic-pituitary level, by inhibition of the gonadotropin releasing hormone (GnRH) pulse and also at the gonadal level (2,5). Pineal gland germ cell tumors cause sexual precocity by release of human chorionic gonadotropin but the mechanism of precocity is unknown with other lesions. Data from animal models and human studies suggest that there is removal of the gonadotropin inhibition by melatonin leading to precocity or stimulation of hypothalamo-pituitary-gonadal axis via a secretory product analogous to GnRH."*

A number of very recent studies of nurses working shifts compared to nurses not working shifts have failed to show an increased risk of breast cancer or even a difference in melatonin production. This is not surprising when we note that, in the modern society, everyone is getting a large dose of light at night. This wasn't the case when the early nurses' studies were done.

I will delay citing the various studies that support the "melatonin hypothesis" as a significant cause of breast cancer until Chapter 17A.

CHAPTER 2A

Light and Sleep

The study of sleep continues to attract more attention, with more than five thousand technical papers having been published in the first five months of 2014. On the other hand, the public continues to treat sleep as something to do when there is nothing more interesting or important to do than sleep.

Light from Electronic Devices

The invasion of the bedroom by the mobile electronic device is almost complete. The iPhone, smartphone, and iPad are always within easy reach even when we are sleeping. The glowing screens rich in blue light are a source of serious concern for sleep doctors.

A study at the Lighting Research Center found a two-hour exposure to light from an iPad caused a significant drop in a person's production of melatonin if used in the hours preceding bedtime. While these devices do not seem that bright compared to a light bulb, they are used close to the face and fill a large fraction of the field of view of the eyes.

In response to this problem, Daniel Carome and Vilnis Kubulins at John Carroll University and Photonic Developments LLC have developed a line of filters for mobile devices and TV and computer screens. These screens block light at wavelengths below about 510nm, which eliminates UV and almost all of the melatonin-suppressing light. Because the eye-brain visual system is so adaptable, the average person doesn't even notice the color change caused by the filters.

Changes in Sleep Patterns

Large changes in sleep patterns occur during a person's lifetime. Toddlers (three years old) tend to be mostly morning types with very few night owl types. This pattern tends to reverse as they grow into adolescents. Because of late bedtimes and early school start times, most students suffer from sleep deprivation and daytime sleepiness. Students adopt late bedtimes partly due to as need to do homework and partly by choice. The choice is partly the result of electronic things to do (computer games, texting friends, etc.) that are more fun than sleeping. A study in Australia found that students whose parents set their bedtimes did get more sleep and performed better in school.

One benefit of longer sleep that I had not encountered before regards the frequency of common illnesses in adolescents. One study found longer sleepers had fewer illnesses and school absences than shorter sleepers. This was more evident in boys than in girls.

Fluorescent vs. Incandescent Lighting

An interesting sleep study in Japan used the ninety-four members of a university soccer club as the subjects. They were divided into three groups: controls, a group in which nothing new was introduced, the second group, who had a tryptophan-rich breakfast (melatonin is made from tryptophan) followed by bright sunlight, and the third group, which was the same as the second except that evening light was switched from the normal blue-white fluorescent to low-color temperature (yellow-orange) incandescent lighting. The melatonin level was significantly higher in the third group than in the control group. Because Japanese homes are typically lighted with blue-white fluorescent lighting, the Japanese probably would benefit greatly from use of the low-blue light products we have developed.

CHAPTER 3A

The Remarkable Discovery That Blue Light Suppresses Melatonin

As in all human endeavors, there may be a number of people who claim a discovery. So it is with the discovery of the special sensors in the human eye that control the circadian rhythm. In a 2011 article in *Scientific American* magazine, a different story is told than the one described in the first edition of this book.

Blind mice were observed to still behave as if they knew if it was day or night. The pupils still responded to light even though there was no vision. These mice had been bred to be devoid of the rods and cones needed for vision.

Years earlier the tails of tadpoles had been observed to darken when exposed to light. Cells from the tails were analyzed, and a new compound was isolated that was similar in structure to the opsins (pigments) found in rods and cones. This compound was named *melanopsin*. When the retinas from the mice that were blind but still had a circadian rhythm were analyzed, they found there was melanopsin present in the first layer of the retina. The first layer was composed of ganglion cells, a few of which contained melanopsin. The absorption spectrum of melanopsin peaks in the blue at about 470nm. This is different from the absorption spectrum of the opsins in the rods and cones. It was therefore believed that the circadian rhythm was controlled by the cells containing melanopsin, not the rods and cones. This discovery of previously unknown light-sensitive cells in the retina was a surprise since the retina had been the subject of intensive research for many years. These cells have come to be called *inherently photosensitive retinal ganglion cells,* which is abbreviated as *ipRGC.* (This was well before we had iPhones and iPads.)

One more experiment was needed to confirm that these newly identified ipRGC contrillled the circadian rhythm. Mice that were missing the gene necessary to produce melanopsin were bred and to everyone's surprise, they had a normal circadian rhythm. This suggested the current theory that when the rods and cones detect light, they send a signal to the ganglion cells, which have nerve fibers going to the circadian clock. This would happen primarily when the ganglion cells are missing melanopsin or when the light lacks the blue component that activates the melanopsin. This accounts for the observation that even red light, if bright enough, will cause melatonin suppression. This is thought to be the way in which the rods and cones exercise weak control of the size of the iris when blue light is not present. Exactly how the communication between the rods and cones and the ganglion cells takes place is not yet known. However, it appears to be a weak connection. As with many control systems in the body, this system has a back-up system. .

Whichever account of the discovery of the ipRGC is more valid—the one recounted in the first edition of this book, or the one described in this chapter—will have to be decided by the historians. In any event, it is this discovery that motivates us to provide lighting that does not damage health and to offer protection (amber glasses) when that type of lighting is not available. It was the basis of our work in 2005 to develop light bulbs that don't make blue light and eyeglasses that block blue light and to set up our website, www.lowbluellights.com, where the public can buy these products.

CHAPTER 4A

The Toronto Experiment

To my knowledge no one has repeated the Toronto experiment. That was the 2005 expseriment in which it was shown that wearing amber glasses allowed the subjects in the study to produce melatonin during the night even when exposed to bright lights. The nearest thing is the experiment that uses amber glasses to shift people's circadian rhythm. That confirms that wearing the glasses has the same effect on the body as darkness does. These glasses are described in Chapter 9A.

The use of the amber glasses with patients with bipolar disorder that will be discussed in Chapter 10 also confirms that the amber glasses make the body act as if it is in darkness. Our experiencehelping thousands of customers sleep better also supports the validity of the Toronto experiment.

CHAPTER 5A

How People Study Sleep

Progress in the study of sleep has been advanced by providing new tools to study it, as described in a quote from a paper by M. Dresler and colleagues:

> *"Polysomnography is the gold standard of sleep research, complemented by brain imaging, neuroendocrine testing, genomics and other laboratory measures that can help to create composite biomarkers that allow maximizing the effects of individualized therapies while minimizing adverse effects."*

Polysomnography is the measurement of many vital signs including brain waves while a subject is sleeping in a sleep laboratory. Brain imaging and genomics are the new technologies that are providing new insights into sleep.

CHAPTER 6A

The Problems with Sleeping Pills

America has become the country where every little problem is treated with something you buy at the drugstore. Dry lips? No problem. Smear on something that will help. Dry mouth? We can fix that with "Bioteen." Got a cold? There is no end of things to try. Can't sleep? You need an expensive prescription drug to get the good stuff. There seems to be very little interest in trying to avoid health problems. Even the doctors don't emphasize wellness but treat every condition with the currently popular pill. "Ask your doctor if Amblify is right for you." TV would go broke without the drug companies.

Ambien (Zolpidem) is the most popular sleeping pill. In 2013 more than 60 million prescriptions were written for it in the United States alone. Recently the FDA reduced the recommended dose to half of what it had been. This was very likely motivated by the large number of complaints from people who were arrested for crashing while "sleep driving" or finding they had cooked and eaten a meal while asleep. Many famous people have had misfortunes after taking Ambien. There is now a website—Ambien Outrage—that documents the bad effects, including many deaths and countless injuries. One of the worst cases involved a woman who killed three people while sleep driving after having taken Ambien.

There is probably a legitimate need for sleeping pills, but it seems that they should be used only if everything else fails.

A major side effect of sleeping pills is described in the following from the SHOUSE California Law Group website.

California Vehicle Code 23152(a) VC prohibits driving under the influence of drugs. This law not only applies to illegal drugs but to prescription and over-the-counter drugs as well. DUI Ambien is one way to invite this charge, even if you don't realize that you are, in fact, driving.

DUI Ambien and "Sleep Driving"

"Sleep driving" is defined by the FDA as "driving while not fully awake after ingestion of a sedative-hypnotic product, with no memory of the event." Ambien and other popular sleeping medications like Lunesta, Sonata, and Rozerem are sedative-hypnotic products that can cause this condition.

Sleep driving while under the influence of Ambien or Lunesta occurs after you take the medication, go to sleep, unknowingly wake up (and start sleep-walking) and then drive a car. It's a growing danger, as hundreds of people continue to suffer California DUI Ambien arrests.

Even though sleep driving has become a recognized phenomenon, and akin to sleep-walking, it is nevertheless illegal. If you use Ambien, Lunesta, or any other "sedative-hypnotic" medication and then drive, you face conviction for a California DUI of drugs charge.

FDA Recognizes DUI Ambien may be an "Involuntary" Act

In 2007, the FDA ordered drug companies that manufacture these types of drugs to warn users of the "sleep driving" side effect. This warning comes in two forms: (1) on a clear label on the bottle, and (2) in a product medication guide that accompanies the prescription.

The fact that the FDA took that action is incredibly significant. It demonstrates that this condition is involuntary, which could arguably act as a defense to a California DUI of drugs charge. A California DUI criminalizes the voluntary act of driving while under the influence. It follows that if there's no voluntary act, then there's no criminal culpability.

The fact that sleep driving is involuntary is further corroborated by the evidence that surrounds a typical DUI Ambien arrest...those stopped are often only semiclothed in sleeping attire, disoriented, and/or oblivious to the DUI investigation. But.

Certain Voluntary Acts Negate This Defense to a DUI Ambien Charge

Ignoring warnings or otherwise improperly using Ambien or other sedative-hypnotic products will invalidate this defense. Most of the cases that have been successfully prosecuted involve cases where the defendant

- *Combined Ambien with other drugs and/or alcohol (despite the fact that a "label warning" advised against doing so), and/or*

- *Exceeded the recommended dosage.*

Similarly, many of those who have been arrested for California DUI Ambien or Lunesta include those who

- *Suffer from the "next day" effect—a continued drowsiness after waking up from the drug-induced sleep, or*

- *Took the drug before they got home, hoping it would "kick in" before bedtime.*

Unfortunately, these scenarios subject you to possible conviction for DUI Ambien, as they meet the very definition of a California DUID under California Vehicle Code 23152(a)—driving under the influence of a drug.

The bottom line is this—be very careful when using these extremely potent sleep aids. If you're taking Ambien, Lunesta, or another prescription or over-the-counter sleep medication, always ensure that you're completely alert before driving. It is also a good idea to hide your keys before going to bed.

In an article for The Fix, a website devoted to information on addiction and recovery, writer Allison McCabe describes many aspects to the sleeping pill problem that I had not heard about before. With her permission, I am quoting parts of the article, which was also published in the Huffington Post.

Ambien, a member of the class of medications known as hypnotics, was approved by the FDA in 1992. It was designed for short term use to combat insomnia and was a welcome change from the prevailing sleep aid at the time, Halcion, which had been implicated in psychosis, suicide, and addiction and had been banned in half a dozen countries. Ambien works by activating the neurotransmitter GABA and binding it to the GABA receptors in the same location as the benzodiazepines such as Xanax and Valium. The extra GABA activity triggered by the drug inhibits the neuron activity that is associated with insomnia. In other words, it slows down the brain. Ambien is extremely effective at initiating sleep, usually working within 20 minutes. It does not, however, have an effect on sustaining sleep unless it is taken in the controlled release form.

After its approval, Ambien quickly rose to dominance in the sleep aid market. Travelers swore by it to combat jet lag, and women, who suffer more insomnia than men, bought it in droves. Sanofi, Ambien's French manufacturer, made $2 billion in sales at its peak. In 2007 the generic version of Ambien was released, Zolpidem, and at less than $2 per pill, it still remains one of the most prescribed drugs in America, outselling popular painkillers like Percocet and prescription strength ibuprofen.

Although the Ambien prescribing information warned, in small print, that medications in the hypnotic class had occasional side effects including sleep walking, "abnormal thinking," and "strange behavior," these behaviors were listed as extremely rare, and any anecdotal evidence of "sleep driving," "sleep eating," or "sleep shopping"—all behaviors now associated with Ambien blackouts—were characterized as unusual quirks, or attributed to mixing the medication with alcohol. It wasn't until Patrick Kennedy's 2006 middle-of-the-night car accident and subsequent explanation to arriving officers that he was running late for a vote that the bizarre side effects of Ambien began to receive national attention. Kennedy claimed that he had taken the sleep aid and had no recollection of the events that night.

Shortly after the Kennedy incident, Ambien users sued Sanofi because of bizarre sleep-eating behaviors while on the drugs. According to Susan Chana Lask, attorney for the class action suit, people were eating things like buttered cigarettes and eggs, complete with the shells, while under the influence of Ambien. Lask called people in this state "Ambien zombies." As a result of the lawsuit, and of increasing reports coming in about "sleep driving," the FDA ordered all hypnotics to issue stronger warnings on their labels.

Not everyone who engages in bizarre behavior as a result of taking Ambien ends up in legal trouble. And some people enjoy the high they get from the drug so much that they are willing to overlook the blackouts and negative consequences that result from their drug use. Most recreational users started out taking the drug to treat insomnia, but found that if they fought the drug's sleep-inducing effect, they could get really high. "It's like having that last drink at the bar when you know you should go home—I'd fight the pill's effects and stay up, often telling my friends insane things like how to turn the light in the room into energy, or how paintings of forest scenes on their walls were actually drawings of mermaids bathing themselves in blood," writes one young woman whose addiction to Ambien caused increasingly bizarre and alienating behavior. She continued taking the pill and staying awake regularly until one morning she woke up with two black eyes and a cut across her nose. Her pillows were bloody, and there was a stranger, naked and wrapped in a rug, on her floor. Neither she nor the stranger had any recollection of the events of the previous night. That situation, though jarring, was not enough to get her to give up Ambien; the high was too good. She took a break, but was soon back to taking it regularly, filled with rationalizations for her erratic behavior (All twenty-somethings take drugs!) It wasn't until she was found wandering the Brooklyn streets in the middle of the night, nearly naked, that she was able to give it up for good.

Rapper Eminem, whose albums have titles like "Relapse" and "Recovery," has been open about his battles with prescription drug addiction, including his near overdose on methadone, his relapse, and his eventual detox. He blames Ambien, however, for huge lapses in his memory over five years and an extended period of writer's block. "...a lot of my memory is gone. I don't know if you've ever taken Ambien, but it's kind of a memory-eraser."

Tiger Woods was also famously associated with Ambien when one of his mistresses claimed that she and the golfer would have "crazy Ambien sex." Ambien lessens inhibitions and erases memories, an ideal combination for someone who is cheating on his spouse. The buzz created by the drug appears to enhance sex as well. One woman described feeling "very relaxed and sensual" when she had sex on Ambien. "I suddenly have floaty energy. I am tired, but energetic. It's almost like I'm in a dreamlike state. I might compare it a little to weed, but nothing that I've done really compares, to be honest."

The darker flipside to Ambien's purported sex-enhancing qualities is that it is becoming increasingly used as a date rape drug. In fact, the only case of "sleep-sex" that appeared in a 2008 medical journal review of case reports on Ambien-related sleep behaviors involved the Ambien taker being raped. The same lack of inhibition combined with amnesia that allows people to commit crimes, indulge in dishonest behavior, and have great sex on Ambien is also an ideal formula for a sexual predator. Ambien is also much more widely available and easily accessible than Rohypnol, the drug usually associated with date rape.

Ambien is an effective sleep aid and a huge money maker for its manufacturer. Most people take it as prescribed and treat their insomnia successfully with no problems. But the problems that do occur with the drug are often extreme and tragic, and they seem to be increasing. (These cases only scratch the surface—currently a man in Northern California is using the Ambien defense to fight a charge of second degree sexual abuse of a minor and third degree sexual abuse of a minor. He allegedly molested a ten-year-old girl in April of 2012. He has no recollection of the alleged molestation and a polygraph test supports his claim. His court case is set for March. There is also a whole website, Ambien Outrage, dedicated to making "the public aware of the dangers of Ambien, Ambien CR and Zolpidem." Additionally it maintains a database of "victims of Ambien," those people who have either been harmed or killed by people on Ambien, or who have themselves committed bizarre acts while on Ambien.

In May of last year, the FDA acted again to change the labeling on Ambien, this time lowering the recommended dose and warning people who take the controlled release version that they "should not drive or engage in other activities that require complete mental alertness the day after taking the drug because Zolpidem levels can remain high enough the next day to impair these activities." If the whole idea of taking a sleep aid is to treat insomnia so that you can function more effectively during the day, being instructed to avoid driving and other activities that require mental alertness seems to defeat the purpose of taking the drug in the first place.

The DEA categorizes drugs according to their potential for abuse and addiction. Schedule I drugs are the most likely to be abused, and Schedule V drugs have the least potential for abuse or addiction. Ambien is a schedule IV drug, and can be prescribed and refilled without restriction.

CHAPTER 7A

Sleep and Mental Illness

About the time I was writing (in the first edition) about how bipolar disorder was being treated by "dark therapy," psychiatrist Jim Phelps, MD, was using our amber glasses to treat patients with rapid cycling bipolar disorder (patients change mood from manic to depressed and back to manic frequently). He had the patients put on the amber glasses at 6:00 p.m. and wear them until bedtime and again from when they awakened until 8:00 a.m. This emulated the fourteen hours of darkness that had been demonstrated to stabilize mood in patients with bipolar disorder. Ten of the twelve patients achieved a stable mood. Two dropped out of the study.

Dr. Phelps has an excellent website, www.psycheducation.org, which describes some of the science behind how controlling light helps to avoid or treat mental illness. Many of the customers for our products mention Dr. Phelps and his website.

There is increasing evidence that melatonin can be beneficial in reducing the risk of depression. A very convincing study is titled "Effect of Melatonin on Depressive Symptoms and Anxiety in Patients Undergoing Breast Cancer Surgery: A Randomized, Double-Blind, Placebo-Controlled Trial." In the melatonin-treated group, three of twenty-seven (11 percent) developed depressive symptoms while nine of twenty (45 percent) in the placebo group developed depression. The pills were taken at the same time every day.

The mechanism by which melatonin reduces depression is not clear. However, one clue may be that lack of a strong circadian rhythm is one symptom of depression. Supplying melatonin by mouth at the same time every day was demonstrated years ago to help synchronize the circadian rhythm to clock time. Treating blind people who have this problem of a non-twenty-four-hour circadian rhythm with a new *melatonin agonist* (a substance that acts like melatonin) is currently the subject of an ad campaign (N24) by Vanda, the company that makes the new drug.

The fact that this study by Vanda is using a synthetic melatonin instead of natural melatonin illustrates the problem that in the United States, melatonin is classified as a food supplement and is not under FDA control. This means doctors cannot prescribe melatonin. This allows drug companies to develop these molecules similar to melatonin and get them FDA approved to do the same job that melatonin does. Blind people could get the same benefit from melatonin, according to the earlier studies, but their doctor probably won't know about these benefits, so they will prescribe the expensive, new drug, and medical costs will go up and up. On the other hand, almost all new drugs are developed by the drug companies at their expense, so if these companies didn't have the ability to sell them for a profit, drug research would come to a virtual halt.

Yet another potential benefit of controlling light to shift the circadian rhythm is in treating obsessive-compulsive disorder (OCD). There is evidence that delayed bedtimes increase the risk of mental illness, including OCD. In a case study recently reported, a woman who had a 6:00 a.m. bedtime was greatly helped by advancing her bedtime to midnight with chronotherapy.

CHAPTER 8A

A Safer Method of Treating Seasonal Affective Disorder, SAD

I do not know whether sleep doctors have started using the method of treating SAD suggested in the first edition of this book: having patients put on amber glasses in the early evening to start the flow of melatonin. The validity of the idea, however, is supported by several papers. The first, from 2010, is coauthored by A. Kayumov, who did the study with the amber glasses (see chapter 2: The Toronto Experiment). This new study found that participants who had no discernible peak in melatonin production (i.e., lacked a circadian rhythm) had difficulty falling asleep, had poor sleep quality and displayed borderline depression.

Another study was carried out with eighth-grade students. Half of the students wore amber glasses before and during school hours for a week. Circadian timing was significantly delayed for these students compared to those who did not wear the glasses. This is the opposite of the effect used in the new method of treating SAD. Here the researchers were delaying the setting of the children's internal clocks by not letting the morning light reset their clocks. In trying to prevent SAD, the glasses are put on in the early evening, which is the equivalent of going into darkness and allows the person's body to start making melatonin when it should (i.e., about twelve hours after the eyes were exposed to light in the morning). This experiment demonstrates that wearing the glasses is the equivalent of being exposed to natural darkness and allows manipulation of circadian timing.

A third study found that the circadian rhythm of melatonin production in humans could be moved either forward or backward in time by controlling light exposure in the morning and evening independent of sleep schedule. Orange-tinted glasses (like those available from lowbluelights.com) were used in these experiments.

The results of the experiments described here point up the basic problem caused by electric lights. We are:

Fighting Our Internal Clock

First thing in the morning when we expose our eyes to light, it resets our circadian clock. Twelve hours later, our circadian clock sends a signal to the pineal gland to start making melatonin. But if we have turned on a light, this sends a conflicting signal, "Don't start." Finally we turn off the light, which tells the pineal gland, "Okay to start making melatonin." Next morning, when we want to wake up, it is still making melatonin. (It can for twelve hours or so.)

We expose out eyes to light, and that shuts off the flow of melatonin and resets the clock. Twelve hours later, our internal clock sends the signal, but we have turned on the light, etc. Every day we are setting the clock ahead in the morning and pushing it back in the evening with artificial light. It's no wonder we have problem with sleep and health. We are is a state of continual jet lag.

CHAPTER 9A

Postpartum Depression (PPD)

The only factual error in the first edition of chapter 12 that I detected is the duration of melatonin flow. It wasn't until after publication of the first edition that a large study found that the flow of melatonin lasts for an average of 11.4 hours, if the subjects are in darkness. (The first edition stated that the flow lasts for nine or ten hours.) The large study found a wide range in both the amount of melatonin produced (some individuals produce as much as ten times the amount produced by other individuals) and the duration of the flow (ranging from seven to fourteen hours).

Studies done since 2008 have pointed to the importance of educating pregnant women to the danger of exposure to light at night if postpartum depression is to be avoided. The problems associated with disruption of the circadian rhythm most frequently occur when women find they need to get up during the night to go to the bathroom and are then exposed to light. For some young women they may not have experienced this need before If she turns on the bathroom light, this may be the start of trouble.

This simple act of throwing the light switch does things to the pregnant woman r and also to her developing baby. First, it stops her pineal gland from making melatonin. Second, it delays the setting of her internal clock if it happens during the first part of the night. It shifts the clock to an earlier hour, if it happens in the second half of the night.

The baby receives melatonin from the mother because the placental barrier that stops many things from crossing to the baby does not block the flow of melatonin. If the start of the flow of melatonin in the mother gets disrupted, this disruption will also occur in the baby's blood. If the mother finds she can't go back to sleep when she goes back to bed, the baby may also experience wakefulness, which may compound the mother's problem. As the baby grows, the mother's need to get up more frequently exacerbates the problem of exposure to light.. The sleeping problems may result in the mother's entire schedule getting way out of whack. If the mother becomes depressed during pregnancy, she is very likely to suffer depression after the baby arrives.

In contrast, if she avoids disruption of her circadian rhythm and keeps her melatonin flowing consistently night after night, both she and her baby are developing their circadian rhythms in synchrony with each other. After the birth, this synchrony between the mother and baby's circadian rhythms can continue in full force. This is because the mother's melatonin appears in her breast milk. This has two important effects: it helps the baby to sleep, and it helps to continue to entrain the baby's circadian rhythm in synchrony with the mother's circadian rhythm. This important aspect of breast feeding is one that I have not seen mentioned before. Learning about these two benefits should help motivate women to avoid disrupting their circadian rhythm by exposure to light at night and to breastfeed their babies.

A recently published review of a number of studies of breast feeding and postpartum depression found clear evidence that breastfeeding reduces the risk for postpartum depression. So it's not just a theory, but borne out by experience.

In other places in this book, I have talked about the benefit of maximizing melatonin by avoiding blue light for a number of hours before bedtime. Here I have been focusing on avoiding blue light when getting up at night. For pregnant women and new mothers this is the number-one most important thing to avoid. However, it is also important to point out that maximizing melatonin by avoiding blue light for a few hours before bedtime is clearly of great value to pregnant women and new mothers. Starting melatonin flow in the early evening makes it easy to fall asleep, and sleep is deeper and more refreshing.

One very powerful benefit of having melatonin present in the body is to protect cells from damage during periods of a lack of oxygen. During the unborn baby's growth, there may be times when the cord is compressed or other reasons that the baby may experience a shortage of oxygen. Melatonin can protect the brain and other organs during those times. Studies with sheep have shown that providing melatonin during birth can protect the offspring from harm from lack of oxygen. Protecting human mothers' eyes from blue light during nighttime labor and delivery to maintain a good supply of natural melatonin is not widely accepted yet, but should be. Don't forget your amber glasses on your way to the hospital!

CHAPTER 10A

The Shift Work Dilemma

Most of the recent studies of shift work find that individuals who have rotating shifts tend not to adapt. That is, while they are working nights during the week, , their circadian rhythm stays the same as it is on the weekend when they keep "norrmal" hours. This strongly suggests that they should try to keep their melatonin flowing during the hours when they sleep on the weekend even while they're working. This may be possible by wearing amber glasses when working at night.

A study in Japan suggests that preserving a shift worker's normal schedule of melatonin production may be easier than I had originally thought. The subjects in the study wore caps with a transparent red visor while working a night shift and found that their melatonin was only reduced by 8 percent compared to those who wore caps with no visor who experienced 52 percent reduction compared to dim light conditions. .

Wearing amber glasses may do a better job in preserving melatonin production, but may attract more unwanted attention than wearing a cap with an opaque visor. If red works, opaque would be at least as good. Not too long ago, nurses wore caps. Perhaps an all-white version of the caps with visors that women navy officers wear would be acceptable.

That wearing a visor should be that successful in preventing melatonin suppression really should not have been surprising. It has been known for many years that the sensors that control the circadian system are located primarily in the lower half of the retina. Most lighting is located in the ceiling. These two facts taken together explain why wearing a visor should work quite well in preserving the melatonin of night shift workers.

CHAPTER 11A

Sunlight and the Human Body

I am not aware of any significant new information regarding this subject.

CHAPTER 12A

Why Don't We Have Any Competition?

We do have a little competition. Some of it comes from Dr. Robert Casper, who was one of the group at the University of Toronto who did the experiment with the amber goggles that proved they protected the volunteers from loss of melatonin, when exposed to light at night. He was interviewed in 2012 by CBC about glasses his group was developing to help people sleep better by preserving their production of melatonin. The glasses are called "ZircLight" and have a filter that blocks out a narrow band between 450 and 480nm. It seems very unlikely that they would really work to preserve melatonin since they would only be eliminating some of the light that suppresses melatonin. The fact that they are not available two years after Dr. Casper discussed their development suggests they probably do not work that well.

Dr. Casper and his colleagues did do a study (published in October 2013) in which nurses working rotating shifts wore the glasses and observed an increase in nocturnal melatonin compared to nurses working the same schedule without the glasses. The paper shows the spectrum of the fluorescent lighting in the hospital and the transmission of the glasses. Contrary to the description in the paper and in the above paragraph, the glasses appear to block all light below about 480nm. The fluorescent lamps have peaks due to mercury emission at about 430 and 490nm and then almost nothing until about 550nm. There is some continuous (in wavelength) light that peaks at about 450nm. The filter knocks out all of this continuum of light: the 430nm peak and most of the 490 peak. Since there is no light from the fluorescents between the 490 peak and the 550 peak, all that is coming through the glasses that will suppress melatonin is part of the 490 peak. So this unique combination of fluorescent lamps and filtering glasses does not, in fact, provide much melatonin-suppressing light.

The question is how unique is this combination of light source and filter? Many of the warmer color fluorescent lamps are like the ones in this study, but the whiter ones have a lot of light between 480 and 530nm that would require filtering to avoid melatonin suppression. LED lights, which are expected to replace fluorescent lamps, have a strong emission peak at about 480nm and not a lot of light between 480 and 530nm, so this scheme might work. The obvious benefit of having to block less of the spectrum would be glasses that don't look weird and therefore would be less likely to be rejected.

New Lighting Products

In a related project, a company called Circadian Technologies has been awarded a large Phase II SBIR (Small Business Independent Research) by the US Department of Health and Human Services (HHS) to develop lighting for use in places where people are working night shift. From the abstract describing the project, it is not clear how much of the spectrum will be blocked, although the description mentions avoiding color distortion. In principle it is possible to produce light that looks white but has little or no light between, say, 430 and 510nm. If an LED that emits at 420 nm and a phosphor that emits beyond 510nm are used, the color of the lamp may not be too bad, although color rendering will be poor.

The principal investigator is Martin Moore-Ede, MD, PhD, who is the CEO of Circadian Technologies and author of more than seventy-eight technical papers. His PhD is from Harvard University, and he taught there for more than twenty years. Dr. Moore-Ede and his team could become serious competition. The good news is that HHS has become interested in the problem of light at night.

Another significant competitor is Lighting Sciences, which is marketing a "Goodnight" bulb that is claimed to help people sleep better. The company claims it produces less blue light. It does, compared to its sister product called "Awake and Alert," which provides extra blue light. The "Goodnight" bulb has about the same fraction of blue (melatonin-suppressing) light (22 percent) as an incandescent bulb, according to our measurements. The good news is that the company is spending a lot of money telling people that they need to cut down on blue light in the evening to improve their sleep. The "Goodnight" bulb is also very expensive, which can only help our sales.

Philips Lighting has introduced the "Hue" lamp, which is an LED bulb in which the color is adjustable using any Internet connection. Dimming the blue and green LEDs can make the color quite red, which should prevent users of the bulb from losing melatonin. This is certainly where the world is going—i.e., to computer-controlled lighting.

It is easy to understand the lighting industry's hesitation to jump into making "healthy" light bulbs, i.e., ones that don't make people sick with deadly diseases. It is a tacit admission that their regular light bulbs are making people sick if used in the manner for which they are intended. This makes ordinary light bulbs a dangerous product from which the public has a right to be protected. The fact that the Danish government paid compensation to a number of nurses who had worked night shift for a long time and developed breast cancer suggests why the lighting companies are slow to get into manufacturing healthier light bulbs.

CHAPTER 13A

How It All Began

In the six years since the first edition of *Great Sleep! Reduced Cancer!* was written, we have continued our efforts to let more people know about the dangers that lie in an ordinary light bulb.

I have been making efforts to interest life and health insurance companies in promoting safe lighting or the use of amber glasses, as they have much to gain by helping people live longer lives free of illness. Once again I have been surprised at the almost total lack of interest. Over the past two years, I have been writing press releases at the rate of two a month (more than forty total), with very little evidence that anyone reads them.

The first edition of this book is selling about a dozen copies a week (eight hundred a year). I believe that this sales pace indicates that the public, at least, has an interest in the topic. (I've written three other books, *Heroes of Cancer Prevention Research,* which sells very slowly, *Pregnant? New Baby? Need Sleep!,* which sells fairly well, and *Another Weight Loss Gimmick? Maybe Not,* which hasn't been out long enough to judge how well it's selling.)

The biggest boost to sales of this book happens when there is a program on a national show that talks about how blue light damages sleep. For example, when a program called "Lights Out" aired on the Canadian Broadcast Company, we got a flurry of orders from Canada.

There is some evidence that the lighting industry is beginning to pay attention. We had a booth at a recent Illuminating Engineering Society meeting, where the speakers talked a lot about blue light and orange glasses. The paper we submitted in support of our poster presentation is printed here. We think lighting for health is the new epoch.

Lighting for Health: The Dawn of a New Epoch

Edward Carome, Richard Hansler, and Vilnis Kubulins
Lighting Innovations Institute, John Carroll University

Abstract

There is increasing evidence reported in detail in the medical literature that low levels of melatonin, the so-called "sleep hormone," increases the incidence of breast and prostate cancer, diabetes, obesity and other serious medical conditions. It has long been known that the time of production of melatonin by the pineal gland can be as long as 11 to 12 hours, i.e., the time spent in darkness by humans as they evolved, but that production stops when the eyes are exposed to light. Thus, since the advent of artificial lighting in developed countries, melatonin production time has been reduced for most people to the time they spend asleep, i.e., to from 6 to 8 hours. When medical researchers proved in 2001 it is mainly blue light at wavelengths below about 520nm that suppresses melatonin production, it opened a way for lighting developers to possibly improve people's health. On the other hand, the new LED white light sources tend to be especially strong in the blue range. LED lighting is being promoted for use throughout the home because of its potentially higher lumen per watt efficacy and much longer life than compact fluorescent lamps and the more widely used incandescent lamps, the production of many of which has been ruled out by the Energy Department. LEDs also form the light sources in the screens of computers and televisions and in the ubiquitous iPads and iPhones and similar hand-held electronic devices that are even taken to bed. Not only has the steadily increasing use of artificial lighting in the evening during the past century possibly contributed to increasing a number of serious medical maladies, but the advent of the use of the blue-light-rich, LED-type lighting may further exacerbate this. In this presentation we consider (a) recent medical research on the health effects of melatonin, (b) how blue light suppresses melatonin production, (c) the intensity levels of blue light in frequently used light sources, and (d) a number of available simple ways to modify lighting to avoid melatonin suppression and possibly improve health.

Introduction

Until now the goal of lighting had been twofold: to enhance human performance and to be aesthetically pleasing. Beginning in the 1990s, scientists have been warning that using ordinary light bulbs at night was increasing the incidence of various very serious illnesses, including breast and prostate cancer. Until 2001 the feeling prevailed that there was not much that could be done about the ill effects, since people were not going to give up using light at night.

In 2001, however, two independent research groups [Brainard 2001, Thapan 2001] reported studies revealing that it is primarily blue light that suppresses melatonin and that there are sensors in the retina (different from the rods and cones) that control the internal clock and the pineal gland that produces melatonin, the so-called "sleep hormone." These newly identified sensors do not contribute to vision (other than partial control of the iris of the eye) and the nerve fibers from them go to the hypothalamus, not the visual cortex.

In 2005 a research group at the University of Toronto [Kayumov 2005] did an experiment in which subjects worked a simulated night shift under bright lights while wearing goggles that blocked light at wavelengths shorter than about 530nm, i.e., the blue part of the visible spectrum. They found that the subjects produced melatonin very much like they had on an earlier night when they were kept in darkness.

Also in 2005, our group at John Carroll University (JCU) developed light bulbs that do not produce blue light and eyeglasses that block blue light [Hansler 2005]. These products were made available at www.lowbluelights.com, operated by a spin-off company, Photonic Developments LLC. These products have helped improve the sleep of 90% of those who have used them. A double blind sleep study based on their use conducted at JCU showed a significant improvement in sleep quality and in mood [Burkhart 2009].

Melatonin Suppression by Home Lighting

Table I. Calculated Percentage of Melatonin Suppressing Light of Various Sources

Source Type	*Percent Melatonin Suppressing Light*	*Lumen Output*
Eccosmart 14W CFL 5000K, 60W Equiv.	*41%*	*922*
GE Soft White 43W Halogen 2700K, 60W Equiv.	*31%*	*812*
GE Soft White 60W Incandescent, 2800K	*29%*	*840*
LS Good Night 12W LED 2500K, 60W Equiv.	*22%*	*918*
LowBlueLights 7W LED 1500 K	*4%*	*371*

In Table I the percent melatonin suppressing light was computed by multiplying the measured output energy versus wavelength curve by a melanopsin absorption versus wavelength curve, i.e., the best fit to the data presented in [Brainard 2001] and [Thapan 2001].

Recent studies [Gooley 2011, Santhi 2012] have determined that typical home artificial lighting levels in the evening are sufficient to produce a significant drop in melatonin production. With the phasing-out of the incandescent lamp, the question arises concerning the newer light sources and their ability to suppress melatonin. Since it is the blue wavelengths that are most effective in suppressing melatonin, measurements have been made of the fraction of the light that is in the blue weighted by the melatonin suppression curve. Table 1 shows the results of measurements of the light output of several types of light bulbs, including those claiming "low" amounts of blue light. That this claim is somewhat overly optimistic is emphasized in Figure 1, where the output spectra of the latter three type lamps listed in Table 1 are plotted, assuming equal incident energy densities. Note that the Lighting Sciences "Good Night" LED lamp emits close to the blue light of a 60 watt incandescent lamp, i.e., a "typical home artificial lighting" source.

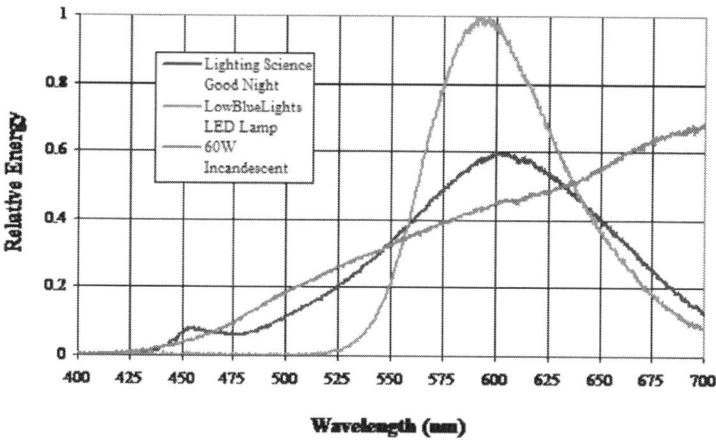

Figure 1. Spectra of three lamps in regions of equal incident energy densities.

The Evidence that Light at Night Damages Health

Animal Studies: *The health effects of light were first observed in small rodents that could be raised in an easily controlled light environment. For example, a study of mice [Nelson 1994] was reported in which female mice were divided into one group raised in 16 hours of darkness and 8 hours of light and a second group raised in the reverse schedule, 16 hours of light and 8 hours of darkness. At eight weeks of age they were injected with a carcinogen. After eight additional weeks it was found that about 90% of the long day mice developed squamous cell carcinoma while none of the short day mice developed tumors.*

An even earlier study [Kothari 1982] in female rats found 95% of the rats developed mammary tumors when given a carcinogen and raised in continuous light compared to 60% that developed tumors when raised in ten hours of light and fourteen hours of darkness. A 1983 study in hamsters [Stanberry 1983] found that eighteen-hour nights increased the time for tumors to start and decreased the rate of growth. They concluded that the quantity, time and duration of melatonin presentation all had an important effect on tumor growth. Many other studies found a similar relationship between hours in darkness, amount of melatonin produced and decrease in the incidence and growth rate of tumors.

Epidemiological Studies: *A study of nurses [Schernhammer 2001] who had worked night shift for many years found they had significantly increased risk for developing breast cancer than nurses who had not worked shifts. A related study [Schernhammer 2009] sampled melatonin in overnight urine in women nurses. They were divided into four groups according to the amount of melatonin measured. Eight years later the incidence of breast cancer was determined. Those with the highest amount of melatonin had about half the incidence of breast cancer as those in the lowest melatonin group. In a related study the nurses with the highest* *amount of melatonin in overnight urine also had a lower incidence of colon cancer.*

A study [Hahn 1991] found that totally blind women had about half the incidence of breast cancer as women with normal vision. In a related study [Flynn-Evans 2009] it was noted there were two types of blind women, those who were totally blind and those who had no vision but whose circadian rhythm (and melatonin production) was controlled by light. Breast cancer incidence was found to be half as great in the totally blind. In totally blind women the flow of melatonin is not diminished by exposure to light.

The incidence of breast cancer is much lower (as much as five times lower) in primitive societies that do not have electric lighting than in the modern western societies [Stevens 2002].

Human Breast Cancer Studies: *Human breast cancers grown as grafts on animals but provided with human blood were found [Blask 2005] to grow rapidly if the blood did not contain melatonin, and slowly or not at all, when the blood contained melatonin.The blood with melatonin was obtained from volunteers during the night and the blood without melatonin was obtained from volunteers during the day or during the night following two-hour exposure to bright light.*

Human Prostate Cancer Studies: *A study [Kubo 2006] of men working night shift showed an increase in the incidence of prostate cancer for night shift workers compared to day shift workers. Men working rotating shifts had the highest incidence. Human prostate cancers grown as grafts on rats but supplied with human blood grew rapidly when the blood lacked melatonin and slowly when the blood contained melatonin.*

Metastasis of Cancer: *Metastasis of cancer to distant sites is the thing that kills most cancer patients, not the original tumor. A breakthrough study [Mao 2012] at Tulane and Thomas Jefferson Medical*

Schools showed that the increased risk of metastasis of both breast cancer and prostate cancer can result from disrupting the circadian (daily) cycle causing loss of melatonin due to exposure to light at night.

The study examined the molecular processes involved in the transition of stable cancer cells into cancer cells capable of moving through the blood stream to distant sites where new tumors can develop. They examined how the presence of various compounds required for the different steps in the process were associated with the presence or absence of melatonin. They looked at this in both cultured cancer cells (both breast cancer and prostate cancer) and also in human cancers grown as grafts on the backs of rats but supplied with human blood. In every case, cancer cells retained a static structure when melatonin was present; however, in the absence of melatonin, the conditions necessary for metastasis to occur were observed.

Seasonal Affective Disorder: *The standard treatment for seasonal affective disorder (SAD), or the winter blues, is to expose the eyes to bright light for about a half an hour first thing in the morning. This will cause the pineal gland to stop making melatonin. It has also been demonstrated to advance the start of the flow of melatonin to an earlier hour in the evening. By starting earlier it finishes its flow earlier, since the pineal gland, even in the blind, can produce melatonin for only 11 to 12 hours, i.e., the time spent in darkness as humans evolved. This solves the problem of too much melatonin in the morning. However, exposing the eyes to light in the evening prevents the flow of melatonin from starting and delays the circadian rhythm, essentially undoing what light in the morning has done. Wearing glasses that block blue light allows the flow to start. The average time for melatonin to flow (if the person is in darkness) is 11.4 hours, according to a recent study [Burgess 2008]. Putting on glasses at 7 p.m. should allow the flow to be over by 7 a.m. This provides a lasting solution to SAD.*

Alzheimer's Disease: *In recent papers from Italy [Polimeni 2014], Russia and the US, scientists have described the possible benefits of melatonin in avoiding and treating Alzheimer's disease. Because* *of exposure to light in the hours before bedtime, most people only make melatonin for 7 or 8 hours a night. A recent study [Lin 2013] of the spinal fluid that bathes the brain suggests this reduction from the maximum of 11 to 12 hours in the time that the pineal gland makes melatonin (and other antioxidants) may increase the probability for the formation of the plaques associated with Alzheimer's disease. Studies in animals and humans [Leston 2009] show that the concentration of melatonin in the spinal fluid is significantly higher than in the blood. Melatonin is thought to be the unique antioxidant that protects the brain from damage by eliminating the free radicals that can damage the brain cells.*

Type 2 Diabetes: *Nurses with the highest melatonin production have about half the type 2 diabetes of those with the lowest melatonin, according to a Harvard study [McMullan 2013]. Quoting from the abstract, "Among participants without diabetes who provided urine and blood samples at baseline in 2000, we identified 370 women who developed type 2 diabetes from 2000–2012 and matched 370 controls using risk-set sampling. Associations between melatonin secretion at baseline and incidence of type 2 diabetes were evaluated with multivariable conditional logistic regression controlling for demographic characteristics, lifestyle habits, measures of sleep quality…" Comparing the results, they found that "Women in the highest category of melatonin secretion had an estimated diabetes incidence rate of 4.27 cases/1000 person-years compared with 9.27 cases/1000 person-years in the lowest category." That is, those with the highest melatonin were less than half as likely to develop Type 2 diabetes as those in the lowest melatonin category.*

Health Benefits of Light

While the psychological benefits of light are recognized by everyone, the actual physiological effect of light has really only been recognized since 2001, when the special sensors in the eye that control the circadian rhythm were identified. The great importance of early morning exposure of the eyes to light in order to reset the circadian clock is still relatively unknown. Providing light rich in the blue component will be a good starting point for the lighting industry. Studies at Rensselaer, GE Lighting, Philips, Lighting Science and Photonic Developments are beginning to provide specially designed lamps with extra blue light for this purpose. Studies in nursing homes [Figueiro 2013] are showing that providing higher levels of light during the daytime results in better sleep at night.

The ideal light source of the future will be one that can change its spectral content with the time of day. During the day it will be a white source, rich in blue wavelengths, and at night it will be devoid of blue light but providing all the other colors. Because of the extremely long lifetime of LEDs, it may be possible for some applications to do away with the idea of an easily replaceable bulb in favor of different designs. The switch from day to night lighting may be as simple as a mechanically operated switch, by a remote control, by an internal clock, or a signal from the provider of the electricity.

Having light sources to use at night that do not disrupt the circadian rhythm is especially important for pregnant women and those with new babies [Hansler 2013]. Sleep is difficult enough to get when there is a baby in the house without this unnecessary disruption from exposure to ordinary lighting during the night.

On the other hand, during the day and under special conditions, recent studies [Sahin 2013] have demonstrated that both daytime and nighttime exposure to blue light is effective in improving human performance on tasks requiring alertness. Instead of turning to caffeine for a boost, exposure to light rich in the blue wavelengths provides a drug-free alternative.

Conclusion

The new epoch in lighting in which the health effects of light become the number one concern is not here yet. But, in step with the introduction of LED lighting, it will very likely be making rapid progress in the very near future.

References

Blask DE, Brainard GC, Dauchy RT, Hanifin JP, Davidson LK, Krause JA, Sauer LA, Rivera-Bermudez MA, Dubocovich ML, Jasser SA, Lynch DT, Rollag MD, Zalatan F, "Melatonin-depleted blood from premenopausal women exposed to light at night stimulates growth of human breast cancer xenografts in nude rats," Cancer Res **65***: 11174–84 (2005).*

Burgess HJ, Fogg LF, "Individual differences in the amount and timing of salivary melatonin secretion," PloS One **3***: 8 (2008).*

Burkhart K, Phelps JR, "Amber lenses to block blue light and improve sleep: a randomized trial," Chronobiol Int **26***:1602–12 (2009).*

Brainard GC, Hanifin JP, Greeson JM, Byrne B, Glickman G, Gerner E, Rollag MD, "Action spectrum for melatonin regulation in humans: evidence for a novel circadian photoreceptor," J Neurosci **15***: 6405–12 (2001).*

Figueiro MG, Lesniak NZ, Rea MS, "Implications of controlled short-wavelength light exposure for sleep in older adults," BMC Res Notes **4***: 334 (2011).*

Flynn-Evans EE, Stevens RG, Tabandeh H, Schernhammer ES, Lockley SW, "Total visual blindness is protective against breast cancer," Cancer Causes Control **20***: 1753–6 (2009).*

Gooley JJ, Chamberlain K, Smith KA, Khalsa SB, Rajaratnam SM, Van Reen E, Zeitzer JM, Czeisler CA, Lockley SW, "Exposure to room light before bedtime suppresses melatonin onset and shortens melatonin duration in humans," J Clin Endocrinol Metab **96***: 2010–2098 (2010).*

Hahn RA, "Profound bilateral blindness and the incidence of breast cancer," *Epidemiology* **2**: 208–10 (1991).

Hansler RL, "Pregnant? New Baby? Need Sleep" (Amazon) (2014).

Hansler R, Carome E., Kubulins V, www.lowbluelights.com.

Kayumov L, Casper RF, Hawa RJ, Perelman B, Chung SA, Sokalsky S, Shapiro CM, "Blocking low-wavelength light prevents nocturnal melatonin suppression with no adverse effect on performance during simulated shift work," J Clin Endocrinol Metab. **90***:2755–61 (2005).*

Kubo T, Ozasa K, Mikami K, Wakai K, Fujino Y, Watanabe Y, Miki T, Nakao M, Hayashi K, Suzuki K, Mori M, Washio M, Sakauchi F, Ito Y, Yoshimura T, Tamakoshi A, "Prospective cohort study of the risk of prostate cancer among rotating-shift workers: findings from the Japan collaborative cohort study," Am J Epidemiol **164***: 549–55 (2006).*

Kothari LS, Shah PN, Mhatre MC, "Effect of continuous light on the incidence of 9,10-dimethyl-1,2-benzanthracene induced mammary tumors in female Holtzman rats," Cancer Lett **16***: 313–7 (1982).*

Leston J, Harthé C, Brun J, Mottolese C, Mertens P, Sindou M, Claustrat B, "Melatonin is released in the third ventricle in humans. A study in movement disorders," Neurosci Lett **469***: 294–7 (2010).*

Lin L, Huang QX, Yang SS, Chu J, Wang JZ, Tian Q, "Melatonin in Alzheimer's disease," Int J Mol Sci **14***: 14575–93 (2013).*

Mao L, Dauchy RT, Blask DE, Slakey LM, Xiang S, Yuan L, Dauchy EM, Shan B, Brainard GC, Hanifin JP, Frasch T, Duplessis TT, Hill SM, "Photoperiodic effects on tumor development and immune function," Mol Endocrinol **26***:1808–20 (2012).*

Nelson RJ, Blom JM, "Photoperiodic effects on tumor development and immune function," Bio Rhythms **9***: 233–49 (1994).*

Polimeni G, Esposito E, Bevelacqua V, Guarneri C, Cuzzocrea S, "Role of melatonin supplementation in neurodegenerative disorders," Front Biosci (Landmark Ed) **19***: 429–46 (2014).*

Sahin L, Figueiro MG, "Alerting effects of short-wavelength (blue) and long-wavelength (red) lights in the afternoon," Physiol Behav 116–117: 1–7 (2013).

Santhi N, Thorne HC, van der Veen DR, Johnsen S, Mills SL, Hommes V, Schlangen LJ, Archer SN, Dijk DJ, "The spectral composition of evening light and individual differences in the suppression of melatonin and delay of sleep in humans," J Pineal Res **53***: 47–59 (2012).*

Schernhammer ES, Laden F, Speizer FE, Willett WC, Hunter DJ, Kawachi I, Colditz GA, "Rotating night shifts and risk of breast cancer in women participating in the nurses' health study," J Natl Cancer Inst **93***: 1563–8 (2001).*

Schernhammer ES, Hankinson SE, "Urinary melatonin levels and postmenopausal breast cancer risk in the Nurses' Health Study cohort," Cancer Epidemiol Biomarkers Prev **18***: 74–9 (2009).*

Stanberry LR, Das Gupta TK, Beattie CW, "Photoperiodic control of melanoma growth in hamsters: influence of pinealectomy and melatonin," Endocrinology **113***: 469–75 (1983).*

Stevens RG, Brainard GC, Blask DE, Lockley SW, Motta ME, "Adverse health effects of nighttime lighting: comments on American Medical Association policy statement," Am J Prev Med **45***: 343–6 (2013).*

Stevens RG, "Lighting during the day and night: possible impact on risk of breast cancer," Neuro Endocrinol Lett **23***: 57–60 (2002).*

Thapan K, Arendt J, Skene D, "An action spectrum for melatonin suppression: evidence for a novel non-rod, non-cone photoreceptor system in humans," J Physiol **585***: 261–267 (2001).*

CHAPTER 14A

Examining the Evidence That Controlling Light Can Cut the Risk of Cancer

The first edition of *Great Sleep! Reduced Cancer!* was published in 2008, so the references cited here are mostly from that year through early 2014. Nothing in current literature suggests that we are on the wrong track. Rather, the evidence keeps growing that maximizing melatonin has more benefits than previously realized.

Some of the recent studies about the benefits of maximizing melatonin include the following:

2007—R. J. Reiter

"Light at Night, Chronodisruption, Melatonin Suppression, and Cancer Risk: A Review"

They state, "For years it was assumed that polluting the daily dark period with light was inconsequential in terms of animal/human physiology. That assumption, however, has proven incorrect." They state that the result is cancer initiation and growth. They point to epidemiological studies that show that the following cancers are more frequent due to light at night and chronodisruption: breast, prostate, endometrial, and colorectal. Mechanisms by which melatonin suppression can enhance cancer have been proposed, but explanations as to how chronodisruption might do this are less clear. The researchers suggest that other diseases may also result from exposure to light at night.

This paper was written in connection with a talk by Reiter at a symposium sponsored by the NewYork Academy of Science that was attended by my colleague Dr. Edward Carome. Dr. Blask also gave a similar paper describing the bad effects of using ordinary light at night. Unfortunately, the media in general have ignored this information, and the general public continues using light at night as if there were no problem.

2007—Vunogradova (from V.Anisimov's Lab):

"Effect of Light Regimens and Melatonin on Homeostasis, Life Span, and Spontaneous Tumorigenesis in Female Rats"

The researchers observed that continuous light or natural light (northwest of Russia) accelerated aging and tumor genesis compared to the standard twelve hours of light, twelve hours of dark. Melatonin given to the rats at night in their drinking water prevented the negative effects. In 2008 the researchers published a second study, this time in male rats, in which they observed the same effects.

2008—I. Kloog

"Light at Night Co-Distributes with Incident Breast Cancer but Not Lung Cancer in the Female Population of Israel"

Nighttime satellite images were used to estimate light at night levels in 147 communities in Israel. Breast cancer and lung cancer incidence for these communities was collected. A strong positive association was found between light intensity and breast cancer rate but not lung cancer rate. A 73 percent higher breast cancer incidence was found in the highest intensity community than in the lowest.

The majority of breast cancers are stimulated by estrogen, and melatonin (which is suppressed by light) guards against estrogen. Neither is true of lung cancer.

2008—V. Srinivasan

"Therapeutic Actions of Melatonin in Cancer: Possible Mechanism"

This study describes how melatonin blocks the conversion of linoleic acid to 1-Hode, a mitogenic (causing cell division) compound. It also inhibits the growth of prostate tumors by activation of MT1 receptors. Melatonin prevents creation of cancer by its antioxidant, immunostimulating, and apoptotic (causing programmed cell death) properties. Melatonin also augments the cancer-killing action of natural killer cells.

2008—A. Kerklinjger-Gruchala

"Low Estradiol Levels in Women of Reproductive Age Having Low Sleep Variation"

The researchers concluded that women who slept regular hours had a much lower (60 percent) production of estradiol. High levels of estradiol have been demonstrated to increase the risk of breast cancer.

This study offers another example of why putting on amber glasses at about the same time in the evening and exposing the eyes to light at about the same time in the morning may possibly be much more important than when you actually sleep.

2008—A. V. Panchenko, N. N. Petrishchev, I. M. Kvetnoĭ, and V. N. Anisimov

"Colon Carcinogenesis in Rats vs. Variable Light"

> *This abstract describing a paper in the Russian journal Vopr Onkol from Anisimov's lab in Russia is very clear and won't benefit from my paraphrasing it.*

Abstract

The effect of lighting and melatonin treatment on 1,2 dimethylhydrazine (DMH)-induced colon carcinogenesis was investigated in rats. There was a direct correlation between constant lighting, on the one hand, and the rate of the process, on the other, and an inverse one between light deprivation and melatonin treatment. That presented as changes in rate of tumorigenesis, number of tumors per animal, adenocarcinoma cell differentiation grade, invasiveness, and proliferative rate. Our results point to light duration as a significant factor of colorectal cancer progression.

2009—A. Korkmaz

"Role of Melatonin in the Epigenetic Regulation of Breast Cancer"

This paper describes, in a highly technical manner, five ways in which melatonin affects the gene environment (that's what *epigenetic* means) in highly beneficial ways.

2009—R. G. Stevens

"Electric Light Causes Cancer? Surely You're Joking, Mr. Stevens"

In the twenty-two years since Stevens introduced the "Melatonin Hypothesis," the evidence has accumulated that indeed, electric light causes cancer, at least breast and prostate cancer. How much longer will it take before somebody does something about it?

In 2005 we, at John Carroll University, did do something about it; we developed lights that won't cause cancer and glasses that will protect against cancer. Strangely (to me) the scientists writing all these papers don't seem that interested. They seem to want to keep studying the problem rather than trying to solve it.

2009—M. Alpert

"Nighttime Use of Special Spectacles or Light Bulbs That Block Blue Light May Reduce the Risk of Cancer."

This was how we, at John Carroll University, introduced the solution to the problem (low blue light bulbs and blue blocking glasses). The only response from the medical community we noted was a letter in *Medical Hypotheses* by Erren and Reiter, who said, "Preventing cancers caused by chronodisruption: blocking blue light alone is not likely to do the trick."

2009—R. D. Stevens (originator of the "Melatonin Hypothesis" in 1987)

"Working against Our Endogenous Circadian Clock: Breast Cancer and Electric Lighting in the Modern World"

Quoting from the abstract, "A new avenue of research has been one function of circadian genes and whether these are related to breast cancer risk. In particular, a length variant of Per3 (5-VNTR) has been associated with increased risk in young women, and this same 5-VNTR variant has also been found to predict morning diurnal type and shorter sleep duration compared to the 4-VNTR variant. An important question is how an effect of light-at-night (LAN) exposure on breast cancer risk might be modified by polymorphisms and/or epigenetic alterations in the circadian genes, and conversely whether light-at-night exposure (e.g., shift work) can induce deleterious epigenetic changes in these genes."

2009—D. E. Blask

"Melatonin, Sleep Disturbance, and Cancer Risk"

This paper was published in a journal that reports primarily on sleep research. This article discusses how melatonin, sleep, and cancer are interrelated. Blask notes that independent of melatonin, quality sleep enhances the immune system. He concludes, "The mutual reinforcement of interacting circadian rhythms of melatonin production, the sleep/wake cycle and immune function may indicate a new role for undisturbed, high quality sleep, and perhaps even more importantly, uninterrupted darkness, as a previously unappreciated endogenous mechanism of cancer prevention."

2009—D. E. Blask

"Circadian Stage-Dependent Inhibition of Human Breast Cancer Metabolism and Growth by the Nocturnal Melatonin Signal: Consequences of Its Disruption by Light at Night in Rats and Women"

This work is an extension of the work reported at length in the first edition of this book on the 2005 study by the same authors. A press release by the head of the National Institute of Environmental Health Science pointed out the significance of this study in explaining how light exposure at night increased the risk of breast cancer. The 2009 paper looked at some mechanisms that include inhibition of linoleic acid uptake, which results in it being metabolized into a cancer-inducing compound (13-HODE). The number of the negative mechanisms increased in parallel with the intensity of the melatonin-suppressing light. Exposure to even dim light prevents the normal circadian rhythm. Blask and his associates conclude with the statement, "This biological mechanism may partially explain the higher risk of breast and other cancers in women working rotating night shifts and possibly others [author's note; i.e., "all of us"] who also experience prolonged exposure to light at night."

2009—E. S. Schernhammer

"Dietary Correlates of Urinary 6-Sulfatoxymelatonin Concentrations in the Nurses' Health Study Cohorts"

The researchers found that the only food that showed an effect on melatonin was red meat. This suggests one mechanism that might explain the observation made earlier by Schernhammer's study that eating red meat increases the risk of breast cancer. One could ask the question "What do light at night and red meat have in common?" Answer: "They both suppress melatonin production and increase the risk of breast cancer." They probably have another thing in common. Most women are not aware of either fact.

2009—E. E. Flynn-Evans (one of Schernhammer's group)

"Total Visual Blindness Is Protective against Breast Cancer"

Earlier studies had shown that blind women had a lower incidence of breast cancer. When it was observed that some blind women still had a circadian rhythm that was controlled by light, the question arose, do they have a higher incidence of breast cancer than totally blind women? The researchers surveyed 1392 blind women in which there were 66 cases of breast cancer (4.7 percent). The odds ratio for totally blind was 0.43. That is, the totally blind were slightly less than half as likely to develop breast cancer as those blind women whose melatonin production was still controlled by light.

2009—I. Kloog

"Global Co-Distribution of Light at Night (LAN) and Cancers of Prostate, colon, and Lung in Men"

This is a continuation of the work cited earlier in a 2008 paper. Once again the researchers found a strong association between light intensity and prostate and colon cancer but not with lung cancer. Prostate and colon cancers are stimulated by estrogen, which is controlled by melatonin, which is suppressed by exposure to light at night.

2009—K. I. Block

"Making Circadian Cancer Therapy Practical"

Quoting from the abstract, "Practical circadian therapy for the cancer patient involves 3 spheres of intervention-improving lifestyle, optimizing internal biochemical milieu, and adjusting treatment times. Integrating all the above treatment modalities has the potential to improve both the quality of life and disease outcomes in cancer patients." This is the group for which we are providing amber glasses for a clinical trial in which an anticipated outcome will be improved sleep of cancer patients.

2010—R. J. Reiter (who has written more than one thousand papers about melatonin)

"Melatonin: A Multitasking Molecule"

Quoting from the abstract, "These uncommonly complex processes often make it difficult to determine specifically how melatonin functions to exert its obvious actions. What is apparent, however, is that the actions of melatonin contribute to improved cellular and organismal physiology."

2010—L. Mao (member of the team at Tulane University)

"Inhibition of Breast Cancer Cell Invasion by Melatonin Is Mediated through Regulation of the p38 Mitogen-Activated Protein Kinase Signaling Pathway"

Quoting from the abstract, "The pineal gland hormone, melatonin, has been shown by numerous studies to inhibit the proliferation of estrogen receptor α (ERα)-positive breast cancer cell lines. Here, we investigated the role of melatonin in the regulation of breast cancer cell invasion." *Invasion* refers to the ability of cancer to spread to other parts of the body, not simply to grow.

2010—S. Proietti

"Melatonin and Vitamin D3 Synergistically Down-Regulate Akt and MDM2 Leading to TGFβ-1-Dependent Growth Inhibition of Breast Cancer Cells"

Quoting from the abstract, "In MCF-7 breast cancer cells, melatonin together with vitamin D3, induced a synergistic proliferative inhibition (working together inhibit cell growth), with an almost complete cell growth arrest at 144hr." The researchers go on to explain in highly technical words the mechanism by which this occurs. This suggests to me that getting sufficient vitamin D3 is another thing one can do to avoid breast cancer.

2010—M. D. Mediavilla, E. J. Sanchez-Barcelo, D. X. Tan, L. Manchester, R. J. Reiter

"Basic Mechanisms Involved in the Anti-Cancer Effects of Melatonin"

The following abstract from a study in *Current Medicinal Chemistry* is such a good (not too technical) summary of how melatonin works (eleven different ways); I thought it was worth printing the whole abstract. *Apoptosis* is cell death, *telomerase activity* is the shortening of the length of DNA strands that is related to aging, *epigenetic* means gene environment, and *angiogenesis* is blood vessel growth, *oncostatic* means cancer arresting and *indoleamine* is internally produced substance, like melatonin.

Abstract

It is commonly accepted that melatonin (N-acetyl-5-methoxytryptamine), the most relevant pineal secretory product, has oncostatic properties in a wide variety of tumors and, especially, in those identified as being hormone dependent. The objective of the present article is to offer a global and integrative view of the mechanisms involved in the oncostatic actions of this indoleamine. Due to the wide spectrum of melatonin's actions, the mechanisms that may be involved in its ability to counteract tumor growth are varied. These include: a) antioxidant effects; b) regulation of the estrogen receptor expression and transactivation; c) modulation of the enzymes involved in the local synthesis of estrogens; d) modulation of cell cycle and induction of apoptosis; e) inhibition of telomerase activity; f) inhibition of metastasis; g) prevention of circadian disruption; h) antiangiogenesis; i) epigenetic effects; j) stimulation of cell differentiation; and k) activation of the immune system.

The data supporting each of these oncostatic actions of melatonin are summarized in this review. Moreover, the list of actions described may not be exhaustive in terms of how melatonin modulates tumor growth.

2011—Higuchi

"Effectiveness of a Red-Visor Cap for Preventing Light-Induced Melatonin Suppression during Simulated Night Work"

Eleven young men tested the visor cap compared to a nonvisor cap.The percent melatonin suppression for men without the visor cap was 52 percent compared to 8 percent for those with the visor cap. Subjective sleepiness was the only observation when using the visor cap.

This study suggests to me that if a red visor cap works to preserve melatonin, then an opaque visor would work at least as well. It also suggests that the main source of melatonin suppression for nurses is the overhead lighting. The working conditions for most night shift workers probably include overhead lighting. Simply wearing that favorite baseball cap will probably preserve melatonin for night shift workers and avoid circadian disruption and increasesed risk of cancer.

2011—A. Grundy

"The Influence of Light at Night Exposure on Melatonin Levels among Canadian Rotating Shift Nurses"

The nurses in this study worked a schedule of two twelve-hour days, two twelve-hour nights, and five days off. The pattern of the nurses' melatonin production did not differ between the two shifts. Looking only at the night shift, higher light level resulted in lower melatonin production. With this schedule there was no indication that the nurses' circadian clocks were reset during night shift work. This means sleep had to occur when melatonin was at a minimum. This would be a case where wearing amber glasses during the night shift would increase the melatonin production and mitigate any increase in the risk of breast cancer.

2011—D. E. Blask

"Circadian Regulation of Molecular, Dietary, and Metabolic Signaling Mechanisms of Human Breast Cancer Growth by the Nocturnal Melatonin Signal and the Consequences of Its Disruption by Light at Night"

This paper describes the anti-invasive/antimetastatic action of melatonin by blockage of p38 phosphorylation. Melatonin also inhibits the growth of human breast cancer by a pathway involving blockage of linoleic acid. The researchers conclude, "Experimental evidence in rats and humans indicating that LAN-induced circadian disruption of the nocturnal melatonin signal activates human breast cancer growth, metabolism, and signaling provides the strongest mechanistic support, thus far, for population and ecological studies demonstrating elevated breast cancer risk in night shift workers and other individuals increasingly exposed to LAN."

2011—V. Kannen

"The Melatonin Action on Stromal Stem Cells within Pericryptal Area in Colon Cancer Model under Constant Light"

The researchers studied the formation (in rodents) of precancerous colon cells following fourteen days of continuous exposure to light. Supplementation with melatonin prevented the formation. This experiment supports Schernhammer's study in which more melatonin in the urine of nurses collected overnight was associated with reduced colon cancer.

2011—K. Ruchter

"Recommendations for the Prevention of Breast Cancer in Shift Workers"

The researchers suggest regular sleep education courses for night shift workers on the prevention of sleep disorders. They note that a person's *chronotype* (inclination to morning type or evening type) is an important predictor for his or her adaptability to shift work.

2011—S. E. Lee

"MicroRNA and Gene Expression Analysis of Melatonin-Exposed Human Breast Cancer Cell Lines Indicating Involvement of the Anticancer Effect"

Quoting from the abstract, "MicroRNAs (miRNAs) are small, non-coding RNAs that play a crucial role in regulation of gene expression. Recent studies have shown that miRNAs implicated in initiation and progression of various human cancers, including breast cancer and also analysis of miRNA expression profiles in cancer, provide new insights into potential mechanisms of carcinogenesis. Our findings suggested that melatonin may modulate miRNA and gene expression as an anticancer mechanism in human breast cancer cells."

2012—J. Wang

"Melatonin Suppresses Migration and Invasion via Inhibition of Oxidative Stress Pathways in Glioma Cells (Brain Cancer)"

This study describes in technical detail the different ways melatonin impedes migration and invasion of brain cancer cells. It concludes, "This suggests a potential therapeutic application of melatonin in the treatment of glioma."

2012—L. Mao

"Circadian Gating of Epithelial-to-Mesenchymal Transition in Breast Cancer Cells via Melatonin-Regulation of GSK3beta"

The spread of cancer from the original site to other organs is what usually kills cancer patients. To spread, breast cancer cells must be in the mesenchymal form. In this study, the researchers demonstrated that melatonin can inhibit this transition. It is thus established that melatonin not only inhibits the growth of breast cancer tumors but also inhibits their spread (metastasis). The researchers also pinpointed the detailed mechanism by which the inhibition occurs. Mao is a member of the group at Tulane University Medical School that is doing such pioneering work on preventing cancer.

2012—E. J. Sanchez-Barcelo

"Breast Cancer Therapy Based on Melatonin"

This study mentions that melatonin has a double action both as a selective estrogen receptor modulator (SERM) and as a selective estrogen enzyme modulator (SEEM). It is thus beneficial either alone or in combination with other anti-estrogen drugs. The study concludes, "Since the strongest suppression of nocturnal melatonin occurs with wavelength light in the blue spectral region, optical and lighting devices filtering the blue light spectrum have been proposed to avoid the risks of light induced suppression of nocturnal melatonin." More than proposed. We have been providing them since 2005.

2012—J. P. Bonde

"Work at Night and Breast Cancer—Report on Evidence-Based Options for Preventive Actions"

This paper reports the recommendations of a panel of experts that convened in Copenhagen in October 2012. They recommended fewer consecutive night shifts for workers and the possible use of red light and reduced light intensity. They recommended more studies of the impact of various shift schedules and type of lighting on breast cancer incidence.. The experts recommended that women who have cancer or have had cancer not work night shift. Use of oral melatonin was not recommended for fear of long-term side effects. Maximizing endogenous (natural) melatonin was not mentioned. There was no mention of our efforts.

2012—M. Dumont

"Melatonin Production and Light Exposure of Rotating Night Workers"

In this study of thirteen rotating shift workers, the researchers found no difference in twenty-four-hour melatonin production whether the subjects were working day or night. Apparently melatonin production continued during the night when the people worked at night and was therefore lacking when they tried to sleep during the day.

2012—Kucuktula

"Protective Effect of Melatonin against Radiation Induced Nephrotoxicity in Rats"

It is well known that inflammation of the kidneys can be a delayed result of exposure to radiation therapy. Melatonin applied intraperitoneally (injected into the belly) at ten milligrams per kilogram provided protection from damage by 20 Gy radiotherapy in five fractions (treatments).

Makes one wonder why melatonin is not being used routinely before procedures like CAT scans, MRIs, and even mammograms. I suspect it is because nobody has figured out how to make money by doing that.

2012—K. Obayashi

"Positive Effect of Daylight Exposure on Nocturnal Urinary Melatonin Excretion in the Elderly: A Cross-Sectional Analysis of the HELJO-KYO Study"

This study used a cohort of 192 elderly people (mean age 69.9 years). They were exposed to daylight that was at least 1000 lux) in brightness (about like a modern office) for a period that varied between 37 and 124 minutes. Melatonin excretion on the following night was significantly associated with daylight exposure, and the increase from 37 to 124 minutes was associated with a 13 percent increase in melatonin excretion. The mechanism by which longer exposure to bright daylight led to more melatonin excretion is not obvious. A similar increase in melatonin that is associated with exercise is also not understood. Stimulation of the pineal gland during the day may allow it to produce more melatonin during the night. Another theory might be the fatigue of the blue light sensors (in the eyes) during the day makes them less sensitive to the suppressing effect of light at night.

2012—V. N. Anisimov

"Light-at-Night-Induced Circadian Disruption, Cancer, and Aging"

The researchers tested three light regimes on both rats and mice of both sexes. Exposure to constant illumination was followed by accelerated aging and enhanced spontaneous tumorigenesis in female CBA and transgenic HER-2/neu mice. The male and female rats were maintained at various light/dark regimens: standard twelve hours of light and twelve hours of dark [LD], the natural light [NL] of northwestern Russia, constant light [LL], and constant darkness [DD]) from the age of twenty-five days until natural death. The researchers found that exposure to NL and LL regimens accelerated age-related switch-off of the estrous function (fertility in females), induced development of metabolic syndrome and spontaneous tumorigenesis, and shortened life-span both in male and females rats compared to the standard LD regimen. Melatonin given in nocturnal drinking water prevented the adverse effect of the constant illumination (LL) and natural light (NL) regimens on the homeostasis, life-span, and tumor development both in mice and rats. The exposure to the LL regimen accelerated colon carcinogenesis induced by 1,2-dimethylhydrazine (DMH) in rats, whereas the treatment with melatonin alleviated the effects of LL. The maintenance of rats at the DD regimen inhibited DMH-induced carcinogenesis. The LL regimen accelerated, whereas the DD regimen inhibited, both mammary carcinogenesis induced by N-nitrosomethylurea and transplacental carcinogenesis induced by N-nitrosoethylurea in rats. Treatment with melatonin prevented premature aging and tumorigenesis in rodents.

2012—E. J. Sanchez-Barcelo

"Melatonin Uses in Oncology: Breast Cancer Prevention and Reduction of the Side Effects of Chemotherapy and Radiation"

The abstract identifies two areas for application of melatonin: "i) treatments oriented to breast cancer prevention, especially when the risk factors are obesity, steroid hormone treatment, or chronodisruption by exposure to light at night (LAN); ii) treatment of the side effects associated with chemo- or radiotherapy. Because of its SERM (selective estrogen receptor modulators) and SEEM (selective estrogen enzyme modulators) properties, and its virtual absence of contraindications, melatonin could be an excellent adjuvant (additive) with the drugs currently used for breast cancer prevention (antiestrogens and antiaromatases). The antioxidant actions also make melatonin a suitable treatment to reduce oxidative stress associated with chemotherapy, especially with anthracyclines and radiotherapy."

2012—P. Lissoni

"Cancer as the Main Aging Factor for Humans: The Fundamental Role of 5-Methoxy-Tryptamine in Reversal of Cancer-Induced Aging Processes in Metabolic and Immune Reactions by Non-Melatonin Pineal Hormones"

Quoting from the abstract, "The most investigated of the aging factors is represented by 5-methoxy-tryptamine (5-MTT), which may exert antitumor, anticachectic, and immunomodulating effects under experimental conditions, in addition to those effects produced by [melatonin] MLT itself. In an attempt to obtain some preliminary data in human subjects about the potential therapeutic properties of 5-MTT, three different studies of 5-MTT have been carried out in advanced solid tumor patients. The first study of MLT plus 5-MTT included 14 thrombocytopenic cancer patients who did not respond to MLT alone. In the second study we have compared the clinical efficacy of MLT plus 5-MTT in a group of 25 untreatable metastatic cancer patients to the results obtained in a control group of 25 cancer patients receiving MLT alone. Finally, the third study of MLT plus 5-MTT included 14 untreatable metastatic cancer patients who did not respond to MLT alone. In all of these studies, MLT and 5-MTT were given orally at the level of 20 mg/day in the evening and at 5 mg/day during the period of maximum light. A normalization of platelet number was achieved by MLT plus 5-MTT in 5 of 14 (36%) thrombocytopenic cancer patients who did not respond to MLT alone. The percentage of disease control obtained by MLT plus 5-MTT in untreatable metastatic cancer patients was significantly higher than that achieved by MLT alone (15/25 [60%] vs. 8/25 [32%], $P < 0.05$). Finally, the association of 5-MTT with MLT induced disease stabilization in 4 of 14 (29%) untreatable metastatic cancer patients who did not respond to MLT alone."

The term *anticachetcic* means against "wasting away," as in loss of weight, muscle tone, etc., as occurs in prolonged illness.

This study is a reminder of why maximizing natural production of melatonin by the pineal gland is important. There are these other hormones besides melatonin that are beneficial.

2013—Y. I. Zhang

"Protective Effect of Melatonin against Adriamycin-Induced Cardio Toxicity"

This drug is used in chemotherapy for several types of cancer. It is known to sometimes damage the heart. In this study (with rats), the researchers found that administering melatonin along with the Adriamycin prevented damage to the heart.

2013—M. G. Figueiro

"Health Consequences of Shift Work and Implications for Structural Design"

The detrimental effects of rotating shift work are enumerated. Use of light to improve alertness is also discussed.

2013—E. L. Haus

"Shift Work and Cancer Risk: Potential Mechanistic Roles of Circadian Disruption, Light at Night, and Sleep Deprivation"

The researchers mention that the short-term effects of shift work are jet-lag-type symptoms and the long-term effects are weight gain/obesity, metabolic syndrome/type II diabetes, and cardiovascular disease and possibly breast cancer. As possible mechanisms for cancer, they mention repeated disruption of the circadian rhythm, melatonin suppression due to exposure to light at night, sleep-deprivation-caused impairment of the immune system, metabolic changes favoring obesity, and generation of pro-inflammatory reactive oxygen species.

2013—R. G. Stevens

"Breast Cancer and Circadian Disruption from Electric Lighting in the Modern World"

The only thing slightly exciting about this paper is that it is copyrighted by the American Cancer Society. Maybe the society is beginning to take the relationship between light exposure and cancer seriously. There is no new information but simply a compelling summary of all the evidence that using light at night is increasing the incidence of at least breast cancer and very likely prostate cancer and colon cancer.

2013—S. M. Hill

"Age-Related Decline in Melatonin and Its MT1 Receptor Are Associated with Decreased Sensitivity to Melatonin and Enhanced Mammary Tumor Growth"

Hill is a member of Blask's group at Tulane. This study was done with young, adult, and old female Buffalo rats. It was found that melatonin production at the nocturnal peak was 35 percent less in adults and 75 percent less in oldsters than in the young. The ratio of night to day production of melatonin was nineteen in young and seven in old rats. The MT1 melatonin receptor was also diminished in the adult and old rats compared to the young. Breast tumors induced with a carcinogen were observed to grow rapidly in the old rats but not in either the young or adult rats. The researchers conclude, "These data suggest that the observed age-associated enhanced growth of tumors is related to the much reduced levels of melatonin and its receptor in aged animals which reduce the sensitivity of tumors to inhibition by exogenous melatonin."

This is the first time (that the author is aware) that the decline in the melatonin receptors with age has been observed.

2013—R. Glenister

"Therapeutic Actions of Melatonin on Gastrointestinal Cancer Development and Progression"

The production of melatonin in the GI tract is related to food consumption (not light). Melatonin regulates antioxidative processes and improves T-helper cell response. Melatonin is directly involved in preventing tumor initiation, promotion, and progression in cancers of the colon, liver, and pancreas.

2013—A. M. Schroeder

"How to Fix a Broken Clock"

There is growing concern that chronic sleep disruption leads to serious conditions such as diabetes (type 2), cardiovascular disease, and cancer. A poorly functioning circadian system results in misalignments of the timing clocks throughout the body. The authors suggest environmental and lifestyle changes to fix the problem. These include light therapy and scheduled meals, exercise, and sleep.

2013—M. Bracci

"Influence of Night-Shift and Napping at Work on Urinary Melatonin, 17-β-estradiol and Clock Gene Expression in Pre-Menopausal Nurses"

Quoting from the abstract, "This study investigated urinary 6-sulfatoxymelatonin (aMT6s), serum 17-beta-estradiol levels in premenopausal shift nurses at the end of the night-shift compared to a control group of daytime nurses. The shift-work group had significantly lower aMT6s levels than daytime nurses independently of a nap. Night-shift napping significantly influences 17-beta-estradiol levels resulting in higher outcomes in nurses who do not take a nap compared to napping group and daytime workers. Our findings suggest that shift nurses experience changes in aMT6s levels after a night-shift. Napping habits influence 17-beta-estradiol levels at the end of a night-shift. These findings might be related to the increased cancer risk reported in night-shift workers and suggest that a short nap during night-shifts may exert a positive effect."

2013—S. Rabstein

"Night Work and Breast Cancer Estrogen Receptor Status—Results from the German GENICA Study"

Quoting from the abstract, "Here, we explored the association between shift work and breast cancer in subgroups of patients with ER-positive and -negative tumors. In total, 'ever shift work' and 'ever night work' were not associated with an elevated risk of ER-positive or -negative breast tumors. Night work for ≥ 20 years was associated with a significantly elevated risk of ER-negative breast cancer."

This result seems to differ from earlier work that showed an association between light at night and increase in estrogen receptor positive breast cancer. The number of subjects who had worked nights for twenty years was small.

2013—J. J. Kooij

"The Circadian Rhythm in Adult Attention-Deficit/Hyperactivity Disorder; Current State of Affairs"

Etiology of the internal circadian rhythm system, the genetic basis for evening typology, overlap between ADHD symptoms and evening preference (night owl), and risk factors for various chronic health conditions, including metabolic syndrome and cancer, are discussed. According to the researchers, resetting the delayed rhythm involves psychoeducation on sleep hygiene, melatonin in the afternoon or evening, and bright light therapy in the morning.

2013—M. Rondanelli

"Update on the Role of Melatonin in the Prevention of Cancer Tumorigenesis and in the Management of Cancer Correlates, Such as Sleep-Wake and Mood Disturbances: Review and Remarks"

Italy is one of the few countries where melatonin is being used to treat cancer in clinical trials both alone and in combination with chemotherapy. Most trials involve patients who are not responding to conventional treatments, so it is remarkable that considerable benefit has been demonstrated. This paper gathers the results. It suggests further testing is warranted. It provides further evidence that maximizing natural melatonin makes good sense.

2013—E. E. Flynn-Evans

"Shiftwork and Prostate-Specific Antigen (PSA) in the National Health and Nutrition Examination Survey"

This study combined three surveys (2005–2010) that determined PSA for men forty to sixty-five years old who were working nights or rotating shifts or not. Results: "We found a statistically significant, age-adjusted association between current shiftwork and elevated PSA at the 4.0 ng/mL or greater level (odds ratio = 2.48, 95% confidence interval [CI] = 1.08 to 5.70; P = .03)." That is, men working nights or rotating shifts were 2.48 times more likely to have an elevated PSA than men the same age who worked days. Conclusion: "Our data support the notion that sleep or circadian disruption is associated with elevated PSA, indicating that shift working men likely have an increased risk of developing prostate cancer."

2014—R. Ghadari

"Urinary Melatonin Levels and Skin Malignancy"

The twenty-four-hour melatonin excretion was measured for seventy patients with either basal cell (fifty-five patients) or squamous cell (fifteen patients) carcinoma and seventy healthy individuals.The mean level for controls was significantly higher than for those with cancer. Sleep duration for controls was also significantly higher. One might speculate that maximizing melatonin will reduce the risk of skin cancer as well as the other ones we have been discussing. On the other hand, the cancer patients' lower melatonin may be because they are in darkness less because they are not sleeping as much as the controls.

2014—B.V. Jaardim-Perassi

"Effect of Melatonin on Tumor Growth and Angiogenesis in Xenograft Model of Breast Cancer"

Human triple-negative breast cancer cells were implanted on mice. Melatonin was injected daily intraperitoneally (in the belly) one hour before lights off. The size of the tumors was measured weekly. The overall result was that "melatonin treatment showed effectiveness in reducing tumor growth and cell proliferation, as well as in the inhibition of angiogenesis" (*angiogenesis* is the generation of new blood vessels for growing tumors).

2014—F. C. Kelleher

"Circadian Molecular Clocks and Cancer"

Peripheral-cell autonomous circadian clocks exist within every cell of the human body and are comprised of at least twelve genes. These include the basic helix-loop-helix/PAS domain containing transcription factors; Clock, BMal1, and Npas2, which activate transcription of the periodic genes (Per1 and Per2); and cryptochrome genes (Cry1 and Cry2). Mice with mutations in Cryptochrome 1 and 2 are arrhythmic (lack a circadian rhythm), and arrhythmic mice have a faster rate of growth of implanted tumors. Compounds that affect circadian rhythm exist with attendant future therapeutic possibilities.

The findings of this study suggest that having a strong circadian rhythm is the surest way to stay healthy. It's nice to know that there are people out there that understand this stuff. At least some of the names of these clockwork genes are starting to sound familiar.

2014—Papantoniou

"Circadian Variation of Melatonin, Light Exposure, and Diurnal Preference in Day and Night Shift Workers of Both Sexes"

Seventy-five night workers and forty-two day workers provided twenty-four-hour urine samples and wore light-measuring devices. Mean excreted melatonin was lower in night workers, 10.9 vs. 15.4. Lowest values were obtained from night workers with morning preference (larks). Peak melatonin excretion was delayed three hours for night workers. Phase delay was stronger among subjects with higher light-at-night exposure and number of nights worked. Conclusion: "Night shift work affects levels and timing of melatonin production and both parameters may relate to future cancer risk."

2014—C. Ramin (Schernhammer's team)

"Chronotype and Breast Cancer Risk in a Cohort of US Nurses"

No association was found in this study between chronotype and risk of breast cancer; with a possible 27 percent higher risk for those who said they were neither morning type nor evening type compared to those who said they were definitely morning type. There were 72,000 women nurses in the study and 1834 cases of breast cancer.

2014—W.Y. Chen

"A Randomized, Placebo-Controlled Trial of Melatonin on Breast Cancer Survivors: Impact on Sleep, Mood, and Hot Flashes"

The purpose of the study was to examine the effects of melatonin supplementation on sleep, mood, and hot flashes in postmenopausal breast cancer survivors. In a randomized, double-blind, placebo-controlled study, ninety-five postmenopausal women with a prior history of stage 0–III breast cancer who had completed active cancer treatment (including hormonal therapy) were randomly assigned to one of two treatment groups. Forty-eight women received three milligrams of oral melatonin daily, and forty-seven received a placebo daily for four months. Compared to subjects on placebo, subjects randomized to melatonin experienced significantly greater improvements in subjective sleep quality as measured by the PSQI, including domains on sleep quality, daytime dysfunction, and total score. There were no significant differences in measures of depression or hot flashes. This is the first randomized placebo-controlled study among breast cancer survivors to demonstrate that melatonin was associated with an improvement in subjective sleep quality, without any significant adverse effects.

This study at Brigham and Women's Hospital and Harvard Medical School confirms our belief that using our glasses to maximize natural melatonin for cancer survivors makes good sense. As mentioned earlier, we are providing glasses for a study by Dr. Block in Evanston, Illinois, that will hopefully demonstrate the benefit. Our readers don't need any more evidence than the above paper. If the glasses don't help, oral melatonin is available.

CHAPTER 15A

The Next Generation of Light Bulbs

In chapter 16 we talked a bit about how the new epoch in lighting is the development of lighting for health. This means we want lots of blue light in the morning and no blue light in the evening. The "Hue" LED bulb by Philips is one of the early examples. The 7-watt LED available from lowbluelights.com is truly devoid of blue light, but since the light is produced by a phosphor excited by the LED, the other colors are rendered quite faithfully. Because LEDs have such a long life, we feel that the trend will be away from screw-in bulbs and toward lighting modules that will provide better heat sinking (heat removal) and better control of light distribution and that can more easily provide both white light rich in blue and also the low-blue light for use in the evening.

CHAPTER 16A

Testimonials

We continue to receive many notes thanking us for developing this technology and indicating how our products have changed lives. One of the very rewarding aspects of our business is the large number of orders from people who indicated they are returning customers.This is a good measure of the benefit people are getting from improved sleep and health.

As a final word, the best thing our customers can do to help others obtain grease sleep and reduced cancer is to tell their friends and neighbors about our products and how they have improved their lives.

15890615R00110

Made in the USA
Middletown, DE
26 November 2014